Obsessive Compulsive Disorder

Reviews of *Obsessive Compulsive Disorder*

'This is an excellent book – full of helpful hints, advice and inspiration for those who suffer from OCD. The authors resist the temptation to simplify, and succeed in providing an insightful guide to a complex problem.'

DR FRANK TALLIS, Clinical Psychologist
and author of *Understanding Obsessions and Compulsions*

'. . . helpful both to those who suffer from the condition and to those who wish to help but struggle to understand.'

JOAN BOND, Director, TOP UK

Obsessive Compulsive Disorder

Practical, tried-and-tested strategies to overcome OCD

2nd edition

Dr Frederick Toates DPhil, DSc

Reader in Psychobiology at the Open University
Visiting Professor in France, Germany and Sweden

and

Dr Olga Coschug-Toates PhD

Physicist

Foreword by **Padmal de Silva**

CLASS PUBLISHING · LONDON

First published by Thorsons as *Obsessional Thoughts and Behaviour* 1990
Reissued by HarperCollins as *Obsessive Compulsive Disorder* in 1992

The authors and publishers welcome feedback from the users of this book.
Please contact the publishers.

Class Publishing (London) Ltd, Barb House, Barb Mews, London W6 7PA, UK
Telephone: 020 7371 2119
Fax: 020 7371 2878 [International +4420]
Email: post@class.co.uk
Website: www.class.co.uk

The information presented in this book is accurate and current to the best
of the authors' knowledge. The authors and publisher, however, make no
guarantee as to, and assume no responsibility for, the correctness, sufficiency
or completeness of such information or recommendation. The reader is
advised to consult a doctor regarding all aspects of individual health care.

A CIP catalogue record for this book is available from the British Library

ISBN 1 85959 069 1

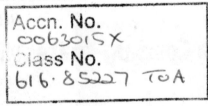
Edited by Gillian Clarke

Designed and typeset by Martin Bristow

Indexed by Val Elliston

Printed and bound in Finland by WS Bookwell, Juva

Contents

Foreword

by **Padmal de Silva**

Obsessive compulsive disorder (OCD), classified in psychiatric thinking as an anxiety disorder, remains a fascinating phenomenon. It is more complicated in its features and presentations than any of the other anxiety disorders – such as agoraphobia or post-traumatic stress disorder – and some aspects of it may seem truly bizarre to those who have no experience of it. Why would someone feel compelled to touch the four walls of a room in a clockwise fashion as soon as he enters it? Why would someone look at an object three times with the right eye, followed by three times with the left eye? Despite excellent scientific and clinical research in the last three decades, OCD continues to fascinate and puzzle.

Much has been written about this disorder, dealing with its nature, its various dimensions and its correlates in recent years. Frederick Toates' book, which was first published in 1990, was one of several books on this subject intended for the general reader. It was, however, different from the others. Here was an author writing about his own experience of suffering from OCD, and also summarising – and commenting on – the scientific literature on the subject. Toates, as a well established and highly accomplished experimental psychologist, wrote on OCD from two vantage points: that of the sufferer, the insider; and that of the scientist who could assess and evaluate the literature. This made his book unique, and it was received with much acclaim.

It is pleasing that a second edition of the book has been prepared. In this edition, written in collaboration with his wife Olga, Toates gives an updated version of his personal story. This is a highly readable and most informative account, a human story told with a frankness that all readers will find touching. In the second part of the book, what is known about OCD and how it is treated is lucidly explained. Even in this part, the personal perspective is not entirely absent; his first-hand experience is there to illuminate, and to illustrate, various points. There is also a wealth of information about many famous people who have had OCD, which further adds to the human interest of the book.

For all these reasons, this excellent new edition deserves to be widely read and widely discussed. I am sure it will be received as a valuable and significant contribution.

Padmal de Silva
Senior Lecturer in Psychology, Institute of Psychiatry,
King's College, University of London;
Consultant Clinical Psychologist,
South London and Maudsley NHS Trust

Foreword to the first edition

by **Professor Hans J Eysenck**

A few years ago, Stuart Sutherland wrote a book entitled *Breakdown* about the psychiatric troubles which all but put an end to his academic career as an experimental psychologist. In this book, Frederick Toates, another well-known experimental psychologist, describes graphically his own troubles with obsessive-compulsive thoughts and ruminations, and gives the reader an opportunity to discover just how debilitating such thoughts can be, and just what they mean in the life of a busy professional man. Both authors clearly needed a lot of courage to disclose their troubles in public, and we owe a debt of gratitude to both for making it much easier for other sufferers to realise that they are not alone with their troubles, and to gain access to professional advice as to what can be done, and what cannot be done, in order to lessen their burden.

One might have thought that psychologists should know enough about the mind not to fall prey to such disorders, but this is not a realistic way of approaching the topic. Just as physicians often fall ill, or have physical diseases, so psychologists and psychiatrists quite frequently fall prey to psychiatric ones – indeed, unkind critics have often suggested that psychiatrists and psychologists frequently take up the study of their subject because they hope to find therein some help for their neuroses! As the ancients used to say: 'Physician – heal thyself!', and the attempts of these two authors to run the gamut of therapies offered on all sides is one of the most interesting aspects of their work. It will certainly be of considerable interest to all those who are suffering from obsessive-compulsive thought disorders, because usually the advice given to them is one-sided, and often based on ignorance rather than on thorough knowledge of what is available. What indeed can psychology do for the sufferer? It would be idle to pretend that we have foolproof methods of treatment which guarantee success, but equally it would be wrong to imagine that nothing can be done. This book discusses in considerable detail the methods used, and what is known about their success, as well as the author's own experiences with them. Anyone suffering from obsessive-compulsive thought disorders, and the attending anxieties and depressions, would be hard put to find a better survey to guide him in this labyrinth. It seems likely that Stuart Sutherland and Frederick Toates are shaping the beginnings of a new tradition in psychological writings, for the benefit of their colleagues as well as of fellow sufferers. Let us hope that this tradition will establish itself quickly, and that other sufferers from psychiatric disorders will come forward to write equally courageous accounts of their sufferings!

H J Eysenck, PhD, DSc
Emeritus Professor of Psychology,
University of London

Preface

In 2001, F.T. was approached by Richard Warner of Class Publishing with a view to issuing a new edition of the book that had first appeared in his name in 1990. F.T. suggested that he should collaborate with his wife on this project. Therefore, Part 2 is a collaborative effort and uses the personal pronoun 'we', whereas Part 1 is the autobiographical account of F.T. and uses 'I'.

Compared with the earlier versions, the emphasis here is more on how you can try to help yourself to cure the disorder. More is now known about treatment, and that is reflected in this edition. References to the material used in writing the book will be available on the Class website: www.class.co.uk.

We would like to express our thanks to Richard Warner, all of the staff at Class Publishing and our editor Gillian Clarke for their outstanding dedication to the task of producing this second edition. We are grateful to Giles Clark of the Open University for advice throughout.

We would love to hear from you, via our publishers at *post@class.co.uk*

Frederick Toates
Olga Coschug-Toates
Milton Keynes 2002

Preface to the first edition

This book describes unwanted, intrusive thoughts and associated compulsive behaviour. The thought that one's hands are contaminated, that one might have done a murder, that two and two might make five, are of this kind. They are irrational in the sense that they are at odds with the rest of the person's lifestyle and purpose in living. I have a peculiar dual interest in this subject, as both a psychologist and as someone with the disorder.

Having had obsessional neurosis over a long period, I have tried a large number of therapeutic techniques. I can't say that any method offers an absolutely reliable cure; one person's cure might only be a source of more suffering to another person. This is therefore specifically *not* a DIY book on how to cure obsessions in twelve easy lessons. If it were claimed to be so, you would rightly ask why I am not able to cure myself. It is perhaps more a 'user's guide' to the obsessional personality and disorder. All that I can offer is the view of an 'expert witness', with some leads that might help both the person with the disorder and those with whom they come into contact. If you have this disorder, I say to you 'You are not alone. In all probability, you are not on the first step towards insanity.' Even that message can be of considerable help to some people. In some cases, medical help proves to be of enormous benefit.

Admitting to mental disorder is rarely easy. Old prejudices die hard, even in the progressive circles of academia. Thus, for no entirely convincing or well thought-out reason, I was very reluctant to go public on this subject. However, in 1986, I read a book by a distinguished researcher in this area, Professor Graham Reed, of York University, Canada. So much of what Professor Reed had to say rang true for me, so I wrote to him to report my own observations. Professor Reed replied immediately, describing me as an 'expert witness' and urging me to go public with my story. At first I resisted. I did not look forward to the prospect of walking down the street mentally naked; neither did I want to provoke the ruminations. However, on reflection, I felt convinced that I had a useful contribution to make, and hence wrote the present book. The first draft of it almost succeeded in omitting from the autobiographical section any reference to sex, thereby possibly implying that I had led a life of celibacy. It was soon pointed out that this was intellectually somewhat dishonest and from this criticism arose the somewhat more frank final version, published in 1990.

By all estimates, literally millions of people in the UK and USA and elsewhere are suffering from this condition, yet many think they are quite alone in their bizarre disorder. Countless people are spending their days washing their hands, checking gas-taps and wondering why two and two make four. Now is the time to come out of the closet! I hope that my going public will help you.

I thank a number of people who have helped greatly in various direct and indirect ways in the production of this book. Julia Adams, Margaret Adolphus, Hans Eysenck, Graham Reed, Padmal de Silva and Madeline Watson read one or more versions, and their comments were of great assistance. An Open University student of mine, Maureen Blandy, pointed me towards the work of George Borrow.

Sometimes, as I ruminated endlessly over the exact choice of words, the music of Fauré, Mozart and Vivaldi, as well as Smokey Robinson, The Beach Boys and The Lettermen, not only helped to maintain my spirits but also gave me a standard of perfectionism to emulate. Finally, my students gave me much inspiration.

Frederick Toates

Part 1
Autobiographical sketch

1
Home in Histon

*'It is by studying little things that we attain the great art of having
as little misery and as much happiness as possible.'*
SAMUEL JOHNSON

At the time I am talking about, Histon was a small village, four miles
from Cambridge. Living there were 'true villagers' and a few 'out-
siders': a Pole and people from the surrounding villages. All the true
villagers knew one another. The village sat between two very different
cultures: on one side the dreaming spires of Cambridge University
and, on the other side, the wild open fens. The academic tradition of
Newton and Russell was far removed from the fen life of Willingham
and Over.

I was born in Histon on 23 October 1943. My parents reflected, to
some extent, the two cultures. Though not a bad pupil, my father had
left school at 14 to work for the Chivers family, whereas my mother
had been brilliant at school in Cambridge, and earned a mention in *The
Times*. The young Minnie Jean Maxim, as she was then called, came to
work as a research chemist at Chivers, where my parents met.
Intellectually and culturally they were very different, but much in love,
with my father having dashing good looks.

In terms of income, we were working class, but we had a middle-
class streak on my mother's side. My mother appreciated Handel's
Messiah; my father had preferred motorbikes and amateur boxing.
I had one sibling, a sister, Mary, six years older than me.

I had a number of fears as a child. Burglary was rare in 1949 but
the prospect still bothered me. I tried to estimate what the chances were
of our home being broken into. Suppose that intruders started at one
end of the village and worked their way house by house. How long
would it be until they got to us? I was frightened of the dark, making
shapes out of shadows on the wall and hiding my face under the sheets.
In spite of all the love and security at home, here were the possible signs
of trouble. However, it is known that fears and rituals are common in
many children, so we cannot place too much weight upon such

evidence. Some relief from the fear of the dark was afforded by fantasy; night after night I imagined the bed to be the cockpit of an aircraft in which I was the pilot, accompanied by an ever-faithful co-pilot named Doedie. We flew for miles over the fens of East Anglia, never crashing once; our control was perfect.

There was some neuroticism in the family. My paternal grandmother could be described as 'highly strung', as could my father, who suffered from spells of depression. These were never serious enough to be incapacitating or to merit seeking medical help. My impression is that we have more than the average share of fears and mild phobias in the family. My father was asthmatic, and hay fever is well represented. I recall my mother 'coming over funny' at the sight of liver in the larder, and my sister being petrified by a spider. The house in which I grew up was cold in winter but the atmosphere was one of unambiguous security. Only twice did I see angry words exchanged between my parents and they seemed to be over matters of triviality. I was encouraged, and received devotion from them. I was fortunate to grow up in a secure matrix of wider family relationships; aunts, uncles and grandparents were all nearby and there was much contact.

School exposed me further to the two cultures: children from the fens spoke one way and those whose parents were associated with the University spoke a rather different English. A rich variety of expressions was acquired at school and taken home; not all of them were either fully understood by me or approved of by my parents. In spite of his own Cambridgeshire accent, my father made it clear that I was expected to speak correctly, using my friend Robert as an example. He added that in later life I would be laughed at if I spoke fen-English. This was all said in a fairly kind, or at least unintimidating, manner. There was the implicit assumption that good speaking was associated with good and morally desirable behaviour. So I was gently cultivated into some of the more easily acquired habits of the middle class. I was sent to piano lessons, but the teacher soon discovered that such talents as I might have possessed were not of a musical kind.

Life was somewhat straight, even Victorian and Calvinist. We were discouraged from displaying strong emotion. On one occasion we were on our way to Heathrow to watch the planes and, to my delight, a Lockheed Constellation coming in to land skimmed low over the bus. I was told not to get overexcited in public. Social respectability, hard work, impeccable manners and correctness of behaviour were emphasised. Taste in clothes was distinctly conservative. The model of behaviour that I acquired from my father was predominantly one of respectability and integrity, with a tendency towards conformity and deference to authority. There was a 'they' out there who generally knew best. On the rare occasions when we visited a café, there was some pressure for all of us to order the same dish, in order not to be difficult. However, my father had a threshold of intolerance, albeit a high one: he could be stubborn when on rare occasions someone was perceived to be trying to get the better of him.

Honesty in dealing with money was especially firmly emphasised, as was the undesirability of asking what things cost or mentioning a person's income. My father was generous with money but parsimonious with natural resources: we were always being instructed to switch lights off wherever possible. He was a 'green' years before the term came into vogue. When making tea for two, he would measure out exactly two cupfuls of water and boil just that amount.

On visiting my father in hospital, my mother issued instructions on correct behaviour: always to stand up when a doctor or nurse came over. At all times, the restrained use of the personal pronouns 'he' or 'she' in the presence of the person concerned was emphasised, the logic of which I had some difficulty understanding.

Not perhaps showing great originality, but certainly sincerity, I informed my parents of a burning ambition to become an engine driver. If I couldn't achieve that, then I wanted some other job on the railways – 'any job, even Swank's, when he retires'. 'Swank', a well-known village character, was the level-crossing keeper.

Hard work, though seen as a virtue by the family, was not always to be viewed as an unqualified pleasure. One day, my father and I were walking through the main street and passed the time of day with some men digging a trench to lay sewage pipes. They were sweating profusely. Looking back, my father pointed to them and said quietly '. . . that is the fate that awaits people who don't try hard at school. But if you do well, nice clean office jobs are available.' All this had the effect of giving me an awareness of social class, but certainly put no pressure on me. It was not said in a way likely to intimidate. In any case, we were part of the class that mattered most in a rural community and cut across all other categories: the respectable.

The children of the village discussed their summer holidays and these were used as the index of our parents' status. Our own family's highest aspirations, of a week at Hunstanton or with relatives in London, did not place us near the upper end of the village social scale.

Histon was then dominated by the Chivers family, who were devoutly Christian. The pub, The Railway Vue, was felt to be out of bounds to Chivers employees at lunch time. The family were held in high esteem in the village. It was with great respect that my father would greet 'Mr Stanley', 'Mr Oswald', 'Miss Hope' and 'Mr William'. They were a kindly and paternalistic family on good terms with their employees. The Chivers' orchards provided a means of earning pocket money for the children of the village, myself included, in the fruit-picking season.

Life in Histon was highly predictable. What to our social class was 'dinner' appeared at 1.05 p.m. and 'tea' at 6.05 p.m. Tea was invariably bread and Chivers jam, with the added luxury of Spam at weekends. Each Saturday we caught the bus into Cambridge to do the shopping and visit my grandmother. During the week, the Chivers buzzer was sounded to announce the start or end of work. On hearing the 6 p.m. buzzer, I would race to the end of the road in order to cycle home with my father.

It seemed that we had no enemies. The village behaved like an organic whole, everything ticked smoothly. I was never warned about the dangers of talking to strangers, possibly because there were no strangers in Histon. Everyone seemed to know their role in life, and there was no one to distrust though there was an abundance of trivial gossip. I was made to feel that harm didn't come to someone growing up in that kind of environment. I acquired a naïve and global trust in the goodness and integrity of my fellow humans, which I have found very difficult to refine in the light of experience.

In spite of the security, there was paradoxically also an insecurity instilled in us, in so far as the physical world was concerned. We tried not to sneeze within earshot of my father, because he was sure to ask whether we had caught a cold. We were regularly instructed never to go out with damp hair or without a raincoat, because you can 'so easily catch your death of cold'. On saying something like 'we will go to London in August', my father would invariably reply 'D V – God willing. Don't forget.' The world of people might well have been a safe one in Histon but, outside this shelter, life was dangerous.

I was over-sensitive, wanted to be liked and make a good impression. If I thought I had caused offence, I would ponder, or ruminate, on the issue inordinately. As a joke, I told Frank, our neighbour, that I no longer liked the plums he gave us each year. My father later pointed out that, unlike his brother Jack, a noted village comedian, Frank didn't have a sense of humour, and I should avoid making remarks that might offend. I was shocked. Too shy to go back and explain what I meant, I kept debating in my mind whether he had taken it in good humour, but couldn't convince myself. On being invited to Robert's house when I was about 12 years old, apart from finding his mother very attractive, I was conscious of attempting to do what was socially acceptable. Later I kept trying to recall exactly what words I had used. It worried me that there might be someone in the world who held me in a less-than-good light.

Histon Baptist chapel had been built by the Chivers family and my paternal grandparents were unquestioningly devoted to the Lord. My own parents were not quite so devout, but I was sent to Sunday school each week and taken to the evening service. Sometimes I was allowed to take a book with me in the evening in case the lengthy sermon bored me. I was fascinated by, even awed by, my Aunt Winnie's copy of Bunyan's *Pilgrim's Progress*.

When a distant relative died, it was explained that the body might be dead but the soul departs from it and goes to heaven. This intrigued me and stimulated much thought. Later, when my goldfish died, I gave it a Christian burial in the garden, marking the spot with a cross made from twigs and 'composing' a short requiem, *This little fish is dead*, to the amusement of the grown-ups.

Each summer the Sunday school went on an outing to Hunstanton. This was a major event in the life of the village: the sandcastles, the hard-boiled eggs dropped on the sand, the deck-chairs and their incumbents wearing knotted handkerchiefs on their heads, were immortalised on film for the benefit of future years. I was taken for a ride on a donkey and my father ended up supporting me and, it seemed, the donkey for most of the way.

There was much humour in the village, including the occasional practical joke, which I much enjoyed. In this and other contexts I was, like my father, blessed with a sense of humour. We were sitting one day on my grandfather's lawn and someone walking past stared at us. My grandfather turned to me and in a strong accent said 'Wha's 'e lookin' at? 'E can go and sit on 'isn grass if he wants.' My emerging awareness of social class was such that, in school for some weeks after this, the memory of my grandfather's expression and accent would come into my mind, and it was very difficult to stop laughing out loud.

Sometimes I looked at my picture-books in church, but much of the time I listened to the service, learning the general notions of sin and goodness, heaven and hell. The prospect of hell-fire was to cause me some very real fear both then and in the future; it would doubtless have helped keep me on the straight-and-narrow for the next few years had my social life been such as to permit anything to pull me off.

Then one Sunday – I guess when I was about 11 years of age – something the minister said made me wonder for the first time about where we all came from. If God created the world, who created God? When did time begin? I was of course not the first to wonder along these lines. What was perhaps odd was my intense fear. This was my first experience of something that in adults would be termed 'existential terror' and it made me very uncomfortable. For ages I thought about this issue, of course getting nowhere. I was fascinated by the supernatural; ghost stories both intrigued and terrified me, sometimes literally bringing me to tears. I wondered whether I would suffer damnation if I mistreated one of my pet newts.

School was a mixture of pleasure and pain. I soon showed some of the makings of an intellectual but, being a loner and non-conformist, didn't devote myself sufficiently to the formal curriculum. My mother helped me with French. I loved biology and collected various amphibians and reptiles at home, to the guarded horror of my parents, who were somewhat phobic towards them. I was put in charge of a museum at school, and made myself busy labelling owl pellets. Another great love was chemistry, and my uncle Ron (Maxim) who was a chemist in Cambridge provided me with some surplus equipment. He was a notable East Anglian photographer and had strong connections with the University, a model uncle to me for intellectual development. My solitary pursuit of science grew into a devotion. One concession to normal boyhood was a fascination with model aircraft. I loved putting transfers of insignia on my models, and reflecting upon their historical significance.

Our annual holiday in London gave immense pleasure – the city was full of stimulation. We were very much country folk coming to the big city. Once, shortly after arriving at Liverpool Street Station, we stepped into the road without looking carefully. A passing taxi driver called out to my father 'Watch it, dad! You're not in the country now.'

At school a sense of politics was awakened in me. My parents were Labour voters, though not with great conviction, and I identified with Labour. Once, when I eavesdropped on a conversation, I heard my mother inform my father that she had just been told about the headmaster's support for Labour. This made me happy. Other children in class were also identified by their politics, and we had lively discussions.

By this time my ambition had risen from engine driver to prime minister. I would later settle for either working for the Labour Party or, very much as a third choice, at the Cambridge 'Butlins', the local pejorative term for the civil service offices.

Life seemed simple; there was injustice in the world and only through socialism could riches be directed to those who needed them. I prayed to God for Socialist victories in various elections throughout the world, though I have no reason to suppose that this influenced their outcome. I wrote to the Labour Party for literature and read it avidly. This was where my heart was. I hated football and cricket, being rather hopeless at all sports; I couldn't stand getting dirty!

My thoughts, which were often of a morbid and egocentric nature, were recorded at length in a special book. I was subject to mood swings, my father sometimes asking why I looked so unhappy. Yet the prospect of a political discussion on the radio in the evening would bring great joy – pleasures in Histon for this 12-year-old were nothing if not simple. Friday evening was particularly exciting, because it was then that Freddy Grisewood presented the political discussion programme *Any Questions?*. Innocent situation comedy appealed to me. In those days, my favourite was *Take it from Here*, perhaps partly because it reminded me of neighbours.

I felt intolerant of my father when he disagreed with me, but in retrospect he was so often right. At times I felt the need to be different, to stand out from the crowd, by for example trying to persuade my classmates that I had psychic powers. My grandmother's repeated praise of my red hair might have helped cement the notion that I was, in some important regard, different.

I started to read avidly paperback books about the war, something that my father tried in vain to discourage, regarding this as being psychologically unhealthy. 'Why not do the same things that other children do?' My morbid fascination with the war was often brought into discussions with classmates.

At the age of about 13, I decided to write a book on the case for nationalisation. On the front was pasted a picture of a Western Region express train. Here was the perfect synthesis: the politics of Utopia and railways, a fusion very meaningful to me. With such credentials, why did destiny not lead me into becoming a vicar? I lent the work to my schoolmate Christopher, who in turn showed it to his father, a Conservative. It evoked the comment 'Not bad. At least he is not a Communist.' I then wrote a short book about a traveller in the Soviet

Union, much to the amusement of a gathering of our family in London.

At this early stage there were some clear signs of obsessionality. I was concerned about where I would ultimately be laid to rest, feeling for some inexplicable reason that this should be in the USA. Rumour was that when the daughter of a certain atheistic professor at Cambridge died, she was simply buried in the professor's garden. This image caused me much distress. There was a perfectionist craving for peace and unity, and an intolerance of ambiguity. Ideas needed to be fitted into a whole, a world view, but this was inevitably frustrated time after time. One day a ticket collector at Waterloo railway station was impatient in giving me directions, and for about two days this caused me to ruminate on the wisdom of nationalisation.

During our holidays with my aunt and uncle in London, I spent much time on my own watching trains at Clapham Junction. Southern Region expresses in beautiful green livery rushing past the platform and destined for such exotic-sounding places as Bournemouth put me on a 'high'. The names of their locomotives, *Biggin Hill* and *Howard of Effingham*, the smoke that they belched and the eerie whistles served to enhance the effect. But even in the midst of such excitement there was little escape from chronic worries about the Labour Party; indeed, the positive emotion seemed to trigger the associated doubts. Things wouldn't fit into a happy whole. Would the Gaitskellite right of centre, where I placed myself, be dominated by the left, with their policy of uni-lateral nuclear disarmament? Gaitskell seemed to represent a secure future, but how secure? I worried a lot that automatic, driverless trains would one day be introduced, as the train would lose its romance in the absence of a living being at the controls. Was it worth all this invest-ment of time and emotion in a system that might be so dehumanised?

A somewhat eccentric and insatiable curiosity led me to visit various fringe political and religious organisations in London, the political aspect being much to the disapproval of my father. 'We will go back to Histon at the weekend if you can't behave like other people.' Though deviations from the norms of society were not welcomed, adherence to respectable middle-class behaviour, such as devotion to homework, was met with lavish and sincere praise. I attended a couple of seances at a spiritualist church in London, where I was offered messages, it was said, from a friend of the family who had been killed in World War II. Later, I compared notes with some others present at the seance. For some time after this I was even more than normally afraid to be in the house alone, though I had been somewhat encouraged by a medium telling me that one day I would make a significant contribution to science. Bird-watching was a passion of mine, and my father encouraged this. Each Sunday morning he would take me to the Histon sewage farm, equipped with binoculars and an identification book. I would avidly tick off those that we had seen. Occasionally, Mrs Schicher, a Quaker, took me to a sewage farm at Milton to look for greenshanks and other fascinating species. My parents regarded establishing contact with adults in Cambridge as evidence of great social confidence, but to me it was just normal. School discovered that I had a talent for public speaking and I was invited to address the parent–teacher association on the subject of spotting birds; I loved the limelight.

Aircraft held great fascination for me. I would cycle to Waterbeach to watch the Hunters. The annual Battle of Britain celebrations were a time of great excitement. On one such open day, my father took me for my first flight, a quick 10 shillings' [50p] worth, a thrilling 15-minute trip over Cambridge in a Dragon Rapide.

Usually I spotted trains alone at Cambridge, but sometimes on a Saturday my father would take me to the main Cambridge to London railway line. As a special treat, I was taken to Huntingdon to see expresses go through at high speed, an awe-inspiring afternoon. Then came the climax of my train-spotting career, a trip to Kings Cross as a special birthday present. The loudspeaker announced 'The Flying Scotsman from Edinburgh will shortly be arriving.' My father and I raced to platform 5, just in time. The haunting sound of the A4 cow-whistle was echoing through the tunnel and we could see the light on the front of the engine. I was trembling with excitement. Here was the perfect synthesis: power, beauty, efficiency, patriotism and public enterprise. I looked with awe at the driver and fireman as they brought this fantastic beast to rest.

I was fascinated by the constituencies of Labour MPs, as listed in the Party diary; I learned ('collected in memory') most of these (I had an extremely good memory). Again in terms of collecting, I loved the I Spy books; one had to spot such things as a Dutch barn and a round church. Through the Daily Herald, my parents had purchased the Odham's Encyclopaedia, in 12 handsome maroon volumes. I spent hours poring over their pages, looking up foreign countries, reading about their imports and exports, learning their capital cities.

On reflection, it is easy to identify possible signs of future problems with unwanted thoughts. For instance, I became a devoted collector of stamps, London trolley-bus tickets and cheese labels, acquiring a large number of these labels from various countries. However, my pleasure in the hobby of fromology was contaminated by the fear that the cheese labels would fade in colour. I wrote to an expert to seek advice and he seemed surprised that this should be a matter of concern. 'Maybe they will fade in time, but that will be ages yet.' The dilemma that something worth having was also mortal, even a cheese label, could not be resolved. Its mortality detracted from its value.

I felt a fear of the 'ships that pass in the night' phenomenon. My parents had taken me on holiday to London to stay with my aunt Olive and uncle David. One evening we were walking in the King George Vth Park in Wandsworth, and, as he so often did, my father struck up conversation with a stranger taking his dog for a walk. The man related to us that he had been recently made a widower and asked about Histon and our holiday. After about 20 minutes, by its persistent tugging, the dog persuaded him to continue the walk. I experienced a deep sympathy for this old chap, a feeling of regret that he would probably never again cross my path. How might I be sure of meeting him again? I arrived at a plan, vowing that five minutes each subsequent day would be devoted to reviving and exercising his memory in my mind. This exercise had no compulsive quality about it; it was a voluntary plan of action. In this way, when we returned to London next year, I would be able to wander about the park, go up to him and say hello. I kept up the memory exercise for some weeks but never met him again.

I was excessively fearful and sensitive as a child. Sad movies easily brought me to tears. After hearing the news that Arthur, a neighbour, had died while eating an orange, I later became nervous after picking one up and recalling this. I caused headaches by acquiring food fads, regarding meat eating as being disgusting. Even when persuaded to toy with a small portion of meat, it was vital that the gravy should not be allowed to contaminate the vegetables. I felt the need to be able to categorise and demarcate foods. For example, if I had eaten cracker biscuits from a plate, I did not like fruit to come into contact with the crumbs.

The opposite sex evoked an uncomfortable mixture of desire, tension and confusion. Sex was not discussed at home, so I was left to learn from kids in the street, some of whom were anything but morally respectable. Fantasy played an inordinate role in forming my ideas. I was socially inept and didn't establish normal relationships with members of the opposite sex. Over time, I had crushes on various girls in the village, particularly Margaret, but never dared do much about it. I admired from afar. At best I would ask a good friend to have a word with her and convey my feelings. I felt strong frustration and wondered whether I would ever find a partner.

I had a crush on Barbara, a girl from Girton. In my fantasy, holding and kissing her drove me wild. Her uncle worked in a post office in Cambridge, and I would go in with the excuse of asking the price of sending a letter to somewhere like Canada. One day, we were on the sports field in Histon, and the wind lifted Barbara's skirt. That was awe-inspiring, such an erotic impact; the breathtaking image with its frustrating connotation of unavailability was to trouble me considerably.

I advised a friend that one should not acquire a girlfriend whose parents were in the armed forces (there were several airbases nearby). The logic was simple: the father could be transferred to Hong Kong and thereby take the loved one away.

A thought pattern seemed clearly to be emerging: life was frightening because of its transient aspect and I should try to protect against this in every way. Security and certainty needed to be built into life.

2
Leaving school

'Happiness must be something solid and permanent, without fear
and without uncertainty.'
SAMUEL JOHNSON, *Rasselas*

After taking my O-levels, I left school to pursue a career in engineering science. I entered a traineeship programme with a scientific firm in Cambridge. One day and three evenings per week and in my spare time, I studied for the exams to allow entry to university. Two years after joining them, the firm were to support me at university.

The factory at first came as a shock to a naïve and formally prudish school leaver. Well-worn and finger-printed sets of pornographic postcards were available on the shop floor, to help relieve the monotony. They evoked in me a mixture of self-righteous horror and erotic fascination.

I found some of my tasks quite intellectually fascinating. I recall devising a new method for inspecting the lamps that were destined for a scientific instrument and being warmly praised for my initiative by the foreman.

As a hobby I learned French and German. I had obtained the rudiments of French in school but this was not taught as a living language. So I bought some books and records, and in my spare time buried my head in the two languages. As I cycled to Cambridge I would imagine everyday scenes in France and Germany, and speak the actors' roles to myself. This consolidated my learning. I guess that I must have shown the obsessional trait of persistence, as later in life I was able to lecture to university students in both languages, as well as Danish.

Sex was, as always, a problem. Still socially inept, I found the establishing of relationships an insurmountable burden. My passions were ignited constantly but to no avail. I was concerned lest the girls I desired should fall into habits of impurity with someone else. That they might fall into impurity with me was a prospect that evoked considerably less dread. I was told that Pauline, whom I had long admired from afar, had been seen on King's Parade one night with an undergraduate. I solved some of my discomfort by reasoning that he might have been a theology student and therefore of impeccable morality.

One day I was taken ill with flu and confined to bed. Thoughts of eternal damnation occupied my fever-ridden mind, and I was torn by conflict. Whatever went on behind the cowsheds would have to be incredibly good to run a risk like that. Life without female contact might be frustrating for me but at least I was not risking damnation.

Each Saturday evening I would take the bus into Cambridge to join some of the workers from the factory for a pub crawl. My friends were older than me, and from them I learned the ways of the world; in exchange I offered gems of wisdom on subjects I had studied. I probably bored them with philosophy and the Labour Party. On one such evening, Len, a compulsive womaniser, introduced me to a friend, Jane, in the bar of The Still and Sugarloaf. Jane was considerably older than me, said to know a thing or two, and I soon learned that she lived in a caravan. She asked me to go to her home, so we said goodbye to Len and took a taxi. Although my morals were still in one respect prudish, such prudery concerned the behaviour of other people rather than myself, so I was not unduly disturbed at the prospect before me. It was there in a caravan, with a parrot looking on, that I lost my innocence, never to regain it. I can't say it was fantastic; in fact, I wondered whether that was really what it could be all about. I was terrified afterwards, spending a sleepless night thinking I might have caught some awful disease.

Life at home in Histon was not all cerebral, though most of it was. I avidly collected popular music discs, falling for the group The Lettermen. I bought everything they made, importing it from the USA if necessary. People told me that they sounded morbid. Now, 44 albums and 40 years on, I am still collecting them. Brand loyalty is surely a trait of the obsessional.

The firm wanted me to spend time in Germany to study engineering techniques and write a report for them. In my fantasy world, occasionally a Heidi or Ursula had entered the compartment of my train and I had been able to play the naïve foreigner role to advantage. Germany might provide a good foraging ground. However, on reflection, as I was on the lookout for a girlfriend here, I thought that Germany might disrupt my plans. It wasn't that Cambridge was bad territory; I was just an awfully incompetent forager.

Thoughts of going to university now aroused mixed feelings. I longed for the intellectual stimulation and big-city life, yet the prospect of being away from home created anxiety. I took David, a socialist working in the electronics assembly shop, into my confidence. 'Suppose', I said, 'that I meet a girl at university who lives far away, in Edinburgh or somewhere. What do we do when the university term ends? Would such a relationship be viable?'

David had long been used to my posing what doubtless seemed eccentric and paranoid questions. He gave me a sympathetic hearing and answer. 'Cross that bridge when you come to it. There will be a solution.' But my inability to wait until reaching the bridge before planning the crossing was becoming very apparent. Every important crossing demanded meticulous planning. Each contingency needed debating; something of such monumental importance as finding a girlfriend could not be left to chance. Nothing must cause me to miss out on life.

3
Student life

*'. . . the obsessive may gravitate toward endeavours that affirm an
illusory acquisition of control, and shun "fuzzier" ones. He believes
that he can someday solve, via intellectual effort and ultimate
understanding, the governing laws of the universe.'*
                                    DR ALLAN MALLINGER,
                                The Obsessive's Myth of Control

I went to the City University, London, to study systems science, which
meant a broad introduction to science and engineering. I felt lonely in
the big city but soon settled down. Some good friendships were established with fellow students in my lodgings in Muswell Hill. On learning
that I had gained a place at university, Mr Chivers came to see my parents and offered financial help if this were needed. My father told Mr
Chivers 'He takes after his mother, you know. Not after me!'

Each Wednesday afternoon was free from lectures and tutorials. This
was so that students could play sport but I preferred to join the curious
and morbid in the public gallery at the Old Bailey. I attended the trial
of the Kray brothers and, after a four-hour queue, that of Dr Stephen
Ward, involved in the Profumo scandal. It was exciting to hear the evidence and brush shoulders with the star witnesses, Christine Keeler
and Mandy Rice-Davies – a new source of fantasy.

I went home some weekends to Histon. Once I was waiting at
Cambridge for the train to Histon and a railwayman asked if he could
help me. 'Do you know what has happened to the Histon train?' I asked.
'You don't know? They closed the line last month.' I was shocked and
angry. How could a country perform such an act of stupidity and
vandalism as to close its railways? The cost to the public purse, in terms
of the damage to the environment, extra load on police, ambulance
and fire services, involved in a switch to road transport would be certain
to exceed the so-called subsidy to the railways. I couldn't see the logic
of it then and still can't today.

Within about four months of starting at university my mother was
taken into hospital. One Friday morning, I received a letter from her,

telling me that she was going home that day and looked forward to seeing me. At the end of the day's lectures, I went to Histon. I was in good spirits, uplifted by the contents of the letter. However, Mrs Eden, a neighbour, saw me walking from the bus stop, stopped to offer a lift and reported that my mother was very ill. Surely this couldn't be right: her letter said that she was going home and wanted to see me. I should have read between the lines and judged by the handwriting, but I have never been good at that, tending to see only what I want to see. The neighbour dropped me at the house, and I entered to find my father in the kitchen in a distressed state. 'She is very ill,' he told me.

I went into the living room and spoke to my mother. She was clearly near to death and I couldn't be sure that she even recognised me, though I prefer to think that she did. I came out of the living room and fainted onto the kitchen floor. My father panicked, thinking I had died. I soon got up and he requested that I should go to bed and leave things to him. The next morning Peggy, a neighbour, came into my bedroom to tell me that Mum had died. I cannot recall any further details until that evening, when the vicar came round to comfort us.

My father was shattered by his wife's death. Any faith in God that he had, seemed to be lost. 'Why me?' was a natural reaction. Mum was cremated in Cambridge on the Tuesday, and I left for London that evening. I was given a sympathetic reception back at the university and did well in my end-of-term exams.

This was now the time for finding a serious girlfriend, and I set my mind to the task. I met various nurses, always of high moral standards, who invariably told me disapprovingly of their associates of lower moral standards. Any disapproval I might earlier have shared was now overshadowed by a feeling of immense regret that I hadn't met the associate. This would keep me awake at night sometimes. On one occasion I did sleep with a girl from Wanstead. This was better than the experience in Cambridge but the relationship did not survive.

Then I found myself a girlfriend and this made me even more attached to the big city and the fun of being a student. However, I soon felt a compulsive need to ring up regularly to find out if she was OK. Then, sometimes after finding out that she was well and feeling happy, my memory would play tricks with me; I would need to ring back to make sure that she really was all right. I told myself that there was something strange in her voice. The compulsive feeling that I should phone was at its worst when it was feasible to phone. After midnight, when it would have been too late to phone, the feeling was somewhat less strong. I was very happy in her presence, but as soon as we parted I had awful withdrawal symptoms. There was no momentum in my psychological make-up, no resources to carry me over. We parted after a year.

After my final exams, I flew to America for a long holiday. I stayed most of the time in a YMCA hostel in New York City and travelled around from this base. My night-time reading was *Cybernetics* by Norbert Weiner, a book that I found in the YMCA library. This finally convinced me that my future lay in the application of my knowledge to psychology.

One day I literally bumped into a girl crossing Times Square. I apologised, and she replied 'That's OK – I like your jacket.' This was wonderful: the excitement of a novel city and a new girl. We got closer and closer as the evening drew on, and she explained that she would be leaving New York City the next day by Greyhound bus. We could hardly retire to my room at the YMCA, so we found a cheap hotel and I signed us in as Mr and Mrs Stanford. My new-found friend rang her parents to explain that she wouldn't be home that night. The next morning when we got up I was thrilled, on turning on the TV by chance, to see The Lettermen. We parted after having lunch together and exchanging addresses. I was then overcome with grief; I couldn't just leave a soul like that, and, in tears, something pulled me irresistibly to the bus station. I asked for help in finding her coach but without success. It had just left.

I was sorry to leave America; I had enjoyed my month and had experienced so much. The Bristol Britannia flew me together with my withdrawal symptoms back to Heathrow. Life was a particular agony exactly one week after my chance encounter in Times Square: the passage of a unit of time since a particular event has always assumed a great significance to me. I couldn't play The Lettermen LP that I had been given, because it evoked such nostalgia.

I had been accepted on an MSc course at the City University, as a logical extension of the BSc, and started back at university in October 1966. It was suggested that I might do a project on the application of systems theory to biology, on the control mechanisms of the eye. A combination of systems theory and biology provided a very satisfying level of intellectual stimulation. I read avidly all the available literature and thought laterally about the results. In the end a novel theory of the eye's accommodation (how the lens changes its curvature to adjust to distance) emerged and has subsequently been widely assimilated into the literature. I loved this work and knew that I wanted the future to be connected with biology or psychology.

As a student of City University, I lived in a hall of residence, Northampton Hall, just off Moorgate. It was here that I met Ljiljana, who was from Yugoslavia and working temporarily in Britain. We married in 1967. I didn't think very much about whether I was making the right decision in getting married, which is perhaps odd given the normal obsessional tendency to ruminate interminably over choices. I bought *Teach Yourself Serbo-Croat* and used every spare moment to learn words and phrases.

One Sunday the newspaper carried an article by Stuart Sutherland, Professor of Psychology at Sussex University. Among other things, Stuart suggested that it would be useful for engineers to come into experimental psychology, bringing their systems understanding to behavioural research. This seemed to be just the cue for which I had been waiting. I wrote to him, was given an interview by Keith Oatley and Professor Sutherland, and accepted to do research towards the degree of doctor of philosophy.

None of us could have supposed just how cruelly the peace of that enthusiastic group was to be shattered in the near future. Stuart Sutherland was to suffer a crippling mental breakdown, recorded in detail in his autobiographical book. I was to suffer obsessional illness combined with depression.

The research topic suggested to me for my doctorate was motivation theory, with particular reference to the biological bases of thirst and drinking – why animals eat and drink when they do. I contacted the firm where I had been employed in Cambridge, explaining the situation and my wish to move out of engineering. They generously wished me well in my new career, saying that, if it didn't work out, to let them know. A holiday was now called for.

Ljiljana and I flew to the Croatian capital, Zagreb. Even with an awareness of the danger of clichés, I can say that I fell in love with Yugoslavia. A romantic streak in me felt empathy for the simple peasant lifestyle, though whether I would ever elect to live it remains a moot point. Provided that the people spoke slowly, I could follow a lot of what they were saying. They sometimes laughed at me when I spoke to them, and, not seeing that the content was particularly funny, I assumed that this was a reaction either to my accent or to mistakes. Croatian with its three genders and seven cases presents a rich scope for errors. However, they insisted that it was for neither of those reasons, just that it sounded funny for a foreigner to speak their language. Sometimes they would lure me into saying innocent words such as 'to eat', which sounded like an obscenity the way I pronounced it.

On returning to Brighton, I started as a postgraduate student at Sussex. In London, university had been rather straight and conservative. Sussex was to be neither. I was struck by the sheer volume of hair in the university, hair everywhere and growing in various places and directions. The revolutionary Left was much in evidence in student affairs: Maoism, Trotskyism and Stalinism. This was a very different socialism from the safety of Attlee and Gaitskell. I staged my own revolt by moving much further to the right, an aberration that would be corrected in time.

I was kept extremely busy at Sussex, working long, strange and unsocial hours to fit in with the nocturnal habits of rats. It made for a rich source of intellectual stimulation but hardly promoted marital harmony. I loved the work. I could not imagine any pursuit in life that could give me as much pleasure as this. I would sometimes have pleasant dreams of rats!

I read avidly and was very impressed with the writings of B F Skinner. His optimistic vision of a utopian society that rewarded good behaviour rather than using punishment for misdeeds was attractive to me. It fitted my own belief that there had to be one right solution to the world's problems. Our task was to move, however slowly, towards this solution.

The delight of being at Sussex University was occasionally tempered by obsessional thinking. I used to dread my birthday, because it reminded me that I was getting older. One day I heard a radio broadcast in which an obsessional was describing her inability to accept the finite nature of existence – that we must all, eventually, die. I felt that I was a bit like that, too. Things were, however, very safely within bounds.

I had always suffered from the occasional nightmare and had even been found sleepwalking outside the house in Histon. Now nightmares were more frequent than before. Their content was of a bizarre nature, consisting of such regular themes as torture and reptiles entering the bedroom. Very occasionally, both then and since, a grief theme has been present. A Freudian would have a field day with such events, but I do not subscribe to the school of psychology that attributes specific significance to the content of our dreams.

At the end of my doctorate work, Keith Oatley applied for two years' money, so that I could stay as a research fellow in the area of motivation. Sussex was a stimulating environment in which to do research in psychology. Almost everyone of significance in the subject paid a visit, including B F Skinner. Brighton was a delightful town. I regarded myself as a most fortunate person to be doing exactly what I wanted in life in such surroundings.

Each summer, Ljiljana and I spent about a month in Yugoslavia, and our relatives came over to stay with us. In 1971 two strange things happened to me. We ascended a tower at Zagreb in order to get a view over the whole city. Until then I had experienced no fear of heights. Indeed, only five years earlier, I had positively enjoyed looking at New York City from the top of the Empire State Building. Now I was really frightened and wanted to come down as soon as possible. A few days later, we were flying back to London, a perfectly normal and regular flight, just like one of the many I had experienced. But suddenly I was terrified. My terror was of one thing only – death – the prospect of a crash. I came out in a cold sweat and shook with fear. On getting to Heathrow, I felt that I would never again be able to get into an aircraft.

Unfortunately, after five years, our marriage was near to an end. I had found myself unable to resist the temptations of the swinging sixties and we parted. I met Gill, who announced she was in an open marriage and was a 'swinger type'. This helped to complete my education. Alas, my wife did not share my new-found 'progressive' ideas. I regretted our parting but accepted that it was probably the best solution. It was a divorce not just from a person but from a whole culture as well, and a vacuum was left. Ljiljana returned to Yugoslavia, and, though this time was not easy, I was not left shattered by it. My mind was soon to be occupied with Denmark.

4
Denmark – almost heaven

'Look round and tell me which of your wants is without supply:
if you want nothing, how are you unhappy?'
SAMUEL JOHNSON, *Rasselas*

I felt the wish to travel and experience a new culture. My attention was drawn to a job as assistant professor at Odense University. Feeling myself to be suitable, I wrote off, and with eager anticipation awaited a reply. Academic jobs were easier to find then than now. Nevertheless, career prospects were a serious consideration. After two months I had given up all hope of hearing from Denmark, and started to negotiate a job in West Germany. Then a letter arrived, with an invitation to attend for an interview the next week. I took the ferry, and arrived in Copenhagen at the flat of Inga, a former colleague from Sussex, ready to go the following day to Odense.

Excitement at the prospect of living in this country filled me as I travelled to Odense. I was interviewed and asked to give a lecture, in English, to a student class. Shortly afterwards the professor informed me that the lecture had been well received and that I was offered the job, subject to the formality of senate approval. Words cannot convey my feeling of total and unqualified euphoria!

Having the chance to sit alone and reflect on the decision, in the train from Odense back to Copenhagen, the euphoria grew. It was a beautiful evening and the scent of the breeze through the window could only confirm the mood of pure pleasure. This was truly a 'peak experience'; I felt that I had come a long way from humble beginnings. Now I could exploit singular and selfish ecstasy. There might have been wars and famine in the world but, right now, the fact that these didn't fit into an acceptable overall perspective need not bother me. The world of my primary concerns simply looked and felt good, and for just a little while that was all that mattered.

At Nyborg two Danish men got into the compartment, one somewhat more drunk than the other. They carried on drinking in the train but this didn't seem to affect their ability to speak good English. When the train crossed the Kattegat on the ferry, they invited me to join them in the bar. What a delight was the sea breeze blowing gently across the ferry, and surely no expensive wine had ever tasted quite so good as the cheap label on offer in that bar. On arriving at Copenhagen, the less-drunk asked if I would take care of the more-drunk, while he went to seek help. We propped him up and I stabilised him against a wall until help arrived. A policeman asked if all was well, and I assured him that it was. This was a great introduction to Denmark. We then all parted, after the less-drunk had made me a homosexual proposition. That evening, Inga and I celebrated the good news by going out for a meal.

In the remaining two days of my stay, there was much for me to see in Copenhagen – the zoo, the Tivoli Gardens and, of course, the mermaid in the harbour, intact with head again. The rough and lively harbour bars were a joy to visit, as was Istergade, then the world's pornography centre. This was an erotic eye-opener; the clandestine black-and-white loan-service in the factory at Cambridge had nothing to compare with this Technicolor.

I returned to England in a good mood; withdrawal symptoms were cancelled by the eager anticipation of a new way of life and the practical tasks involved in moving abroad. Odense University telephoned to announce senate approval of my appointment. My thoughts turned to learning to speak Danish, and so I acquired a 'Teach Yourself Danish' course. Over the next few weeks, the record player relayed a set of phrases and stories in Danish; while shaving, cooking and eating, I was incessantly bombarded at each possible moment. I enjoyed these sessions of language absorption, in the company of Linguaphone's Copenhagen family, the Hansens. I soon made good progress in my fifth language. Danish is a relatively easy language to learn, and that wonderful feeling of being able to monitor one's progress was with me as I gained in confidence.

As the date for my departure drew near I worried that something might go wrong. Keith Oatley, my supervisor, gave me advice as best he could, probably feeling that these conversations were taking creative worrying to ridiculous lengths. Would I get my work permit? Would the Danes decline EEC membership and not want foreigners in the country? The work permit arrived safely, just as Keith said it would. And I had not been taken ill at the last minute.

September 1972 saw my departure from England by boat, with all my worldly possessions in three large suitcases. I stopped off briefly in

Odense to organise myself, and then left for a week's holiday in Sweden. The holiday was a delight, but at the end I was glad to board the Stockholm–Copenhagen sleeper to take up residence in Denmark.

The weather was excellent and the suburbs of Copenhagen, their houses flying the red and white Danish flag, and the stirring of activity on a new day, provided a welcome sight in the early morning sun. This country was growing on me fast.

The professor at Odense showed me my office and then we went to the university flat that had been allocated to me. Just a few minutes' walk from the university, it was ample for all requirements. The first day brought an invitation from a lecturer to have an early dinner with him that evening. Before going out, I took a shower in my new-found home, and felt simply ecstatic. How could life have so much to offer? But it was to have still more. Søren W asked me in and opened a bottle of wine. 'Let's drink to your promotion,' he said.

'But, what promotion?'

'They didn't tell you? You have just been made into a full lektor of the university.' Reflecting on Histon and on the university here, I glowed inwardly and raised my glass. Were there no limits to how good life could be?

Søren had an evening engagement and I decided to spend the remainder of the evening wandering around the town centre. On entering a bar, I was recognised by some students who had been at my interview lecture. They invited me to join them for a drink and then took me on to a disco. Whenever I hear Don McLean's 'American Pie', memories of that lovely evening are revived. The taxi taking me home got hopelessly lost in the fog and I was most impressed when, finally arriving at my flat, the driver refused to take any money for the fare. Here was a reminder of the moral scruples of my upbringing. The following night I went out for a meal with Winnie, whom I had met on the ferry and who taught in Odense.

I began work very diligently by starting to prepare lecture notes. When finally convinced that the teaching plans were in order, I turned to research and working on my first book, which had been started at Sussex. The first lecture series was to be given in English, while I was busy working at Danish. The university ran a course 'Danish for foreigners' which I attended, together with twelve others, including a Yugoslav, a German and a Nigerian. Our only common tongue was Danish, and like foreigners everywhere, in our conversations we sought a bond by tending to exaggerate the eccentricities of our host country.

Television helped a lot with the language, because half of the pro-grammes were in English with Danish subtitles. Of the rest, a significant number were German, French or Swedish, so watching TV served as a congenial language laboratory. My German and French improved as well as my Danish. The staff–student liaison body was told by their student representative that my lectures were much appreciated, a tit-bit of nice news relayed to me by Søren A. There were occasional language problems, but for the most part the students understood English well.

Denmark seemed such a small country, almost having the feel of a village about it. I was regularly able to swoon over its glamorous Minister of Education and MP for Odense, Ritt Bjaergaard, shopping in the local supermarket. On writing a letter one day to the Minister of Transport, Jens Kampmann, concerning a traffic scheme, I asked a friend where to obtain the address. 'In the phone-book, under Kampmann' was the answer. So I sent it to his private address and got a hand-written reply from him.

Within about a month of arriving, I was introduced to a research assistant in physiology, named Mette. The following evening, Mette and I visited a disco, where 'good vibes' echoed between us. In the next few weeks I spent little time in my own flat, preferring to be with Mette in her house in Fruens Bøge, a suburb of Odense.

Christmas 1972 brought an invitation to Mette's parents' home in Valby. They lived in a large old house. This was a time for visiting rela-tions, drinking and eating plenty. This is what Danes call *hyggeligt*, a word having no obvious English equivalent but is epitomised by a group of Danes sitting around a fire in a comfortable flat and eating choco-lates. By now I was fairly competent at Danish and could participate in the conversation. In Mette's family, meals were a grand affair, with different glasses for red and white wine.

After Christmas, the family were invited for a big get-together by Mette's grandparents. Drink was flowing freely and the conversation was good. Switching between Danish and English meant that every-one had a turn at exercising their foreign tongue. However, when we were having coffee, something was wrong; I was feeling sad. I had started to think about the killings in Northern Ireland and to compare my lot with that of the rest of the human race. I was not feeling any sort of guilt; hard work had got me to the University. I had no frustra-tion in life, by any flight of the imagination. I had everything that I could have dreamed of. I had no suppressed anger or, if I did, I had suppressed it so well that I knew nothing of it. As an undergraduate, I had read about the ancient philosophers who warned of the perils of pleasure being turned into pain. Samuel Johnson had been eloquent on the same theme, in his classic *Rasselas*, but now all of this was happening to me and it was awful. It was agony.

This was a strange variety of sadness. I excused myself from the table and went into the study. The walls were covered with old family photographs, handsome blond Danes, and as I glanced at them I felt a distinct emotion, perhaps best described by the word 'grief'. But why? I was not grieving for anyone, not even missing anyone. No one had died or gone away. But this did not seem to matter; the object of my grief was the fragility of life, that life is uncertain, that the human condition is a precarious one. How long could the good life last? What had led me to this luxury, while others were being bombed and shot? I was not responsible for their suffering and I was not guilty over it, but I was being powerfully reminded that nothing is certain. These thoughts passed through my mind but words cannot capture the terror that I felt, the fear that one day what is will be no more. Mette was alive and well in the next room but things could be otherwise. She came into the study to see how I was and I burst into tears.

'What's wrong? Have I done something? Has someone offended you?'

I tried to explain that it was because life was so good that I felt so sad, but this inverse logic made little sense to her. How can one explain disembodied grief? What sense does anticipatory grief make? 'What is happening to me?' I asked myself. I had everything that I could possibly dream of. Why was I sad? The paradise of Denmark seemed to be showing its first sign of turning sour.

5
Signs of trouble ahead

'Thus, a dead fly was in my phial, poisoning all the pleasure which I could otherwise have derived from the result of my brain sweat.'
GEORGE BORROW, *Lavengro*

After the new year, we took the train back to Odense. I was sorry to leave Mette's family but looked forward to getting back to the students. The holiday had been mixed; it was mainly good fun and relaxation but had been contaminated by the episode of sadness. I wondered about what had set off this negative reaction but in general life felt very positive.

I was getting better at Danish all the time and took evening classes in sociology where I was able to participate fully in discussions. Being a Copenhagener, Mette occasionally spoke about our moving from small-town Odense but I resisted. Life had just become so good to us and I didn't want any better, at least not yet. I would move to Copenhagen, yes, but not to another country, except perhaps Sweden. She accepted this and stopped talking about moving overseas.

In February 1973, Mette went with her family on a long-arranged skiing trip to Norway. Although it was only for one week, I dreaded the thought of her going. I saw her off on the Copenhagen train, with a lump in my throat. This was like being at a funeral. I felt shattered, scared and alone, but couldn't say exactly why. I had some good friends in the university and in the evening classes. There was nothing concrete to fear or feel sad over. Mette would soon be back. I was not worried that she would leave me for someone else. She was unlikely to come to harm on the gentle slopes of Norway. The job at the university was going brilliantly. But it was like the morbid experience in Valby: the same feeling of grief all over again, as if Mette had died.

Using emotional blackmail, I had tried for some time to persuade Mette to give up smoking, showing the trait well known among obsessionals of trying to reform their loved ones. Mette promised that while in Norway she would make a special effort to give up.

After seeing the train off, I went straight back to work but was unable to concentrate. Proofreading with the secretary, the task assigned for the afternoon, proved impossible. I was desperately fighting back the tears and she could see it. So I went home to weep. On Saturday evening I was invited to dinner with some friends and, not yet having a phone of our own, used theirs to call Norway. Speaking to Mette cheered me up. I felt quite good for the remainder of the week.

Mette returned from Norway, still smoking but looking beautifully brown. We took a taxi from Odense station to our home in Fruens Bøge and it felt so good to be together. Life went on very well for some months, with no abnormal reactions or thoughts.

A year in Denmark passed, and all in all it had been an excellent period. The lectures were well received. The book was with the publishers. I had been back to England to see my father and sister. In a confident mood, I announced that in future all my lectures were to be in Danish. The University agreed that this would be desirable. There was so much to think about and so much to do.

At about this time, I perceived that something strange was starting to happen. While engaged in, say, reading a book or looking out of a train window, unpleasant thoughts were appearing in my consciousness. They concerned tragedy, illness and death, and always had the common theme 'The good life will not last'. At first seldom in their appearance, but getting more and more frequent, these thoughts both depressed and scared me. They detracted from the pleasure of life, contaminating the experience that otherwise was on offer.

There was some continuity from the past in that I had always been a chronic worrier, often seeing particular disasters ahead. Somewhat similar themes had occasionally arisen before but these thoughts were now rather different in form. They were exaggerated, without cause, alien and irrelevant to my activity and plans. They were frequent and insistent. The unwelcome intrusions would have their frightening effect and then go away, to leave me with the thought patterns that I wanted. Some of the intrusions concerned my own vulnerability and mortality, and others concerned Mette, but the general theme was always 'This heaven of Denmark will not last for ever. Doesn't that detract from its current value?'

Typically, thoughts about my current academic pursuit would switch out and my own death would take over for about 30 seconds, sometimes for much longer. Then about ten minutes later, Mette's death would be presented to my consciousness. The obsessional nature of the thoughts was characterised by their taking over, their blocking of my voluntary course of mental activity. The thoughts intruded and threw me off course; I needed to get back into the logical flow of the scientific discourse.

To try quantifying the unquantifiable, I would say that these intrusions both frightened and depressed me in about equal proportions. Sometimes their fear-evoking power was dominant and at other times I would describe them as more depressing or frustrating than frightening.

At times it seemed that specific and appropriate cues triggered the thoughts, such as reading an obituary or seeing a news report on the Vietnam war. More often, they appeared just to be spontaneous or 'free-floating'. My intrusions have never been associated with a standard automatic 'neutralising' thought or ritual (see Chapter 11 for a discussion of neutralising thoughts). The only time that counter-thoughts (i.e. a thought that tries to 'cancel out' the original intrusive thought) have been present is when I have consciously attempted to devise them, and no given counter-thought ever remained in use by me for any substantial length of time because they invariably failed to work.

Sometimes the thoughts suggested no obvious course of action. In such cases, the intrusion of death would take a 'passively associated' form in that I thought of no course of action – mental or physical – to effect in response to it. Simply the certainty and unavoidability of death would occupy me. At other times the thoughts concerned the prospect of a particular mode of death in the near future and urged a course of action to avoid it. Typically I would read about the numbers killed on the road from Copenhagen to Odense, and this would form the principal theme of the spontaneous obsessions for some days. It might lead me to take two buses rather than a bus and taxi (this was before Green awareness). Not wishing to talk about the ruminations, I always found a rational excuse to present to others, such as that there was a paper I had to read and three hours on the train to Copenhagen would allow this.

I experienced inordinate difficulty in arriving at certain decisions, for example buying things in a supermarket. I would select some Israeli oranges, and then imagine that they might have been poisoned, so I would return them to the shelf and select some Chilean grapes. I would then imagine these to have been contaminated by either the CIA or the KGB, according to the current political climate in Chile, and would return my preference to the oranges, and so on. I was scanning for potential disaster. Ironically, I would gladly have eaten Israeli oranges, or Chilean or any other sort of grapes, there and then in the super-market; the worry concerned only the future prospects, the *anticipation* involved in taking them home with me.

My intrusive thoughts stimulated much reasoning that seemed moti-vated by the need to make them less painful but which was invariably fruitless. I would go round the same loops time after time, and always the logic that was presented as the best solution had the same total lack of conviction. You are now 30 years old . . . That's a lot of years . . . You will be only 60 years old when another 30 years elapse . . . It's ages yet. Don't worry. It's so long until you die that, in effect, it's an eternity. But then the inevitable reply would seem to come from another part of my brain: no – it isn't! The last five years appear to have gone quicker than ever. Four times five is 20 and in 20 years' time you will be 50. That's nearer to death than now, by a significant amount. And so it went on; the same fruitless calculations and estimations, the unwanted retort making the situation worse rather than better.

Statistics of accidents were ruminated on at length, as follows. The figures show that so many people are killed each year on the roads. The population of Denmark is around four and a half million. Divide one by the other and then divide by 365 and your chances for today can be calculated. A small chance. Yes, but someone has got to be the one, so why not you or Mette? So it went on and on. No matter what calculation I did the conclusion was always the same: that life is a risk and perfect security cannot be obtained. There was always room for fear, intense fear.

My death-related intrusions didn't conflict with any moral principle; I was not offended by them in any meaningful sense. I didn't consider myself a bad person or a weak one for having them. However, they clearly went against my goals in life – to attain pleasure, to have a wide range of experiences. They were tormenting, interfering with my work; they caused me to cancel journeys. They contaminated the experience of pleasure. In the seventeenth century, John Bunyan compared his intrusions to 'a clog on the leg of a Bird to hinder her from flying', and I could put it no better than that. Life would have been bliss for me with-out these thoughts – everything else was right about my existence. I regarded them simply as an intrusion, like interference on a television screen. I didn't try to interpret any hidden message behind them.

Generally, my intrusions followed a hierarchy; one object of fear would be more or less replaced when a more frightening candidate came along. For example, ferry boats across the Kattegat can suddenly seem much less frightening when someone invites you to fly to New York. In general, I found the arousal of a fear by, for example, a natural reminder, to be much less painful after the fear was no longer the dominant one. Suppose one particular frightening thought were to be toppled from top place by another. It might then feel as if the loser were trying to wrest control back. This was not usually successful, unless new information was obtained to boost the strength of the loser. Such a hierarchy of obsessions, with one being dominant and an apparent competition, is also often seen in subjects where there are multiple distinct obsessions (e.g. cleanliness and checking) rather than one central theme (e.g. death) that comes up in different forms.

I found that when a dominant intrusive theme had been resolved, as very occasionally happened, a glow of euphoria would be experienced and the world would be beautiful and trouble-free. Predictably, the effect was invariably short-lived. A visit to the doctor and reassurance would typify such a situation. This experience is vividly portrayed in the Woody Allen film *Hannah and her Sisters*, where Mr Sachs, played by Allen, leaves the hospital jumping with joy after learning that he does not have a brain tumour. However, he is all too soon stopped in his tracks by the intrusion of the thought that this represents only a temporary stay of execution and death will find him one day.

I must have irritated my doctor with my imaginary illnesses, each of which seemed convincing to me. Sometimes what is good and beautiful in life would be turned into bad. For example, I would touch Mette and this would arouse fear in me of what could happen to her in the future: imagining that wonderful form as no longer a wonderful form was tormenting.

Despite the intrusions, life went on as usual. I didn't tell anyone about them and thought that in time they might go away. The professor was delighted at my teaching in Danish, having attended the first lecture. My ego was increased by his comments. It went up still more when a Bulgarian student stopped me to announce that mine were the first lectures he could understand. 'The way the Danes speak is impossible for a foreigner to understand,' he informed me.

Strange as it might sound, I was still happy most of the time. Even though intrusions came often, 90 per cent of my time was spent with thoughts other than the intrusion. No one at work thought I looked ill, or, as far as I know, perceived that anything was particularly odd about my behaviour. Obsessionals are often inveterate experts at covering their tracks even where overt rituals are concerned. Denmark suited me well. I put a lot of effort into developing a computer model of feeding (one that mimics the processes underlying feeding and offers explanations), working in collaboration with David Booth at Birmingham. This work showed great promise and it was very rewarding for me.

I started to feel homesick for England, a sentiment that was unknown to me during the first year. I would look forward to watching trash on TV just because it was British trash, material that I wouldn't have dreamed of watching in England.

6
Decline

*'I finished dressing and left the room, feeling compelled, however,
as I left it, to touch the lintel of the door. Is it possible, thought I,
that from what I have lately heard the long-forgotten influence
should have possessed me again? but I will not give way to it . . .'*
GEORGE BORROW, *Lavengro*

By November 1973, when I had just turned 30, the ruminations were getting much worse in both intensity and frequency, and I decided to seek help. So bad were they that the term 'intrusion' would be something of a misnomer, as they were rapidly forming the major content of my consciousness. My GP gave a receptive and sympathetic hearing. I was referred to a local psychiatrist, who asked a large number of questions about my life, background and ambition.

I made several further visits and was told that the problem arose from a subconscious fear of losing Mette to another man. The logic seemed odd and somewhat arbitrary to me. I had never once considered the prospect. How did he know it was that? I was told to write down the content of my worry, then tear up the piece of paper so as to exorcise the thought symbolically. Some medicine was prescribed. The psychiatrist's attitude was polite but strictly formal. He was the only person in Denmark to whom I spoke for any length of time using the formal *De* (you) rather than the informal *du*. The tablets worked at first, in that my mood improved, but this was a small mercy since their effect soon wore off. The dose was increased, thereby causing the symptoms of Parkinsonism, an excruciating combination of muscular rigidity and fidgeting. It felt like I imagined a Chinese torture to be. Further tablets were prescribed to take away the symptoms of the first lot. I was getting more and more worried about the future but was still able to function. The country that had offered so much was now turning sour. The intrusions were to become more intense and frequent, and there was no defence. The jolt of the alarm clock in the morning was the most painful event of the day and the evenings were perhaps the least painful.

I then sought help outside conventional medicine. A well-known hypnotist lived in Odense and a meeting with him was arranged. He gave me a demonstration on a willing young subject and I was impressed. I was convinced that he had something to offer when I observed him performing therapy over the telephone to a Swedish air force officer in danger of sliding into alcoholism. However, when he tried the technique on me, it was clear to both of us that I was immune to his words. He didn't charge me anything, saying that he felt the failure was because I was analysing the situation. 'If only you were able to switch off the scientist in you and give yourself to it.'

One night, in desperation, I turned to the Danish equivalent of the Samaritans and was made very welcome in a local church. The pastor put the Christian argument on pain, suffering and death to me but I remained unconvinced. On leaving him, I was told that, despite everything, I still had a warm smile and asked 'Please – try not to lose it'.

Out of the chaos and complexity of mental illness, one certainty emerges: human sympathy and empathy are such that most people want to help. Also, most, irrespective of their expertise or lack of it, irrespective of school or technique, will claim that they can help. I have found very few indeed (possibly only one) who say that they have little or nothing to offer. This does not mean that people are making false claims in order to boost your morale or make money. Some might do just that but I don't think I have met any. The feeling of wanting to help is overwhelming and tends to colour everything. In the case of obsessional neurosis, there is often the feeling that one can treat it by the use of common-sense rationality, or by logical extension of what would be appropriate in treating, say, depression or marital disharmony. Alas, such good intentions might unwittingly make the condition worse.

In addition to the conventional, you are likely to meet the fringe or even crank elements. If my experiences are anything to go by, even a hard-nosed scientist will try almost anything on offer when times are desperate. There lurks the suspicion that even a method that seems nonsensical and scientifically unsound might just work for reasons that we don't yet understand. Even meeting total strangers while travelling, I would at first feel naïvely that they might hold some secret key to understanding life and would be anxious to strike up conversation with them. They seemed to have a mastery over existence that I was lacking; if only they could teach me.

I answered an advertisement in the local newspaper for a new form of therapy. The therapist turned out to be a Russian immigrant who, on learning where I was from, spoke excellent English. 'My method is that you send me a sample of your blood. Prick your finger with a needle, let some blood drip into a small container. Send it to me, I will feel the vibes and transmit a healing signal to match them.' I didn't pursue it.

The transcendental meditation movement was holding a series of lectures in Odense, so I subscribed and was taught meditation. At first an almost drug-like euphoria was obtained, but over a period of daily sessions, the effect wore off. I now suspect that it might (and only *might*) have been worth persisting for longer.

I was sometimes able to reduce very significantly the frequency and particularly the intensity and quality of the intrusions by drinking alcohol, but this of course brought only temporary relief and the after-effects were most unpleasant. Under alcohol, even if the content of the thought was the same, its cutting edge of fear was blunted somewhat. I could have slid into alcoholism but, mercifully, I did not rate the chances very highly and I was spared it. How I was able to resist when the temporary positive effects were so evident, I do not know.

My compulsive behaviour developed at around this time. Sitting on a bus, I would fix on a passenger who had just alighted, and try to hold him in my gaze for as long as possible. If I couldn't hold him until the bus turned the corner, I was worried that this was an omen that tragedy might shortly befall me. Crazy? Irrational? Yes, particularly for a scientist who had hitherto prided himself on the disinterested and objective pursuit of knowledge, but it was compelling. It lasted for some months and then slowly went away.

I found that I had to go to the toilet immediately before a meal; otherwise, I felt the pressure in my bladder would spoil the experience. Whether I had a full bladder or not, had recently been to the toilet or not, I felt compelled to urinate before the meal. I had to be certain that I had fully emptied my bladder, so the visit to the toilet was longer than might be expected. The logic was odd. 'A full bladder would clearly detract from the meal. But you don't have a full bladder. You know you don't. But, if you did, it would detract. I can't eat the meal on the basis of the information that I believe, but I must test the information that I don't believe in case it is true.' Discomfort would distract from a pleasant experience like eating in a Chinese restaurant. It would not be so distracting from a somewhat less desirable activity like marking exam papers, and so then there would be little or no urge to urinate.

I also found myself checking and double-checking that I had switched off electrical equipment, locked doors, etc. I could not resist going back for yet one more 'final' check. This behaviour was about to add to the discomfort of what was to be the worst day of my life until then, as I slipped deeper into depression.

I took the morning train to Svendborg to meet a friend of a friend. Being into alternative medicine, he might just have something to offer. In fact, he couldn't do much but I was well received in his room in a home for retired clergy. Later in the day, he ran (!) with me back to Svendborg station and wished me well. I felt at an all-time low in the train, made worse by a group of lively young students who served as a painful reminder of when times were so infinitely better, at London and Sussex. Could all that pleasure in living really be over for good? How long would this hell last and would I get even worse? I couldn't imagine what it would be like to be in a mood even worse than this. I was now in a state of panic, feeling, I guess, something like the proverbial rat trapped in a corner.

Getting back to Odense at about 8 p.m., I went to the University to make sure that everything was in order. On leaving, I carefully checked that the laboratory equipment had all been switched off, but then went back for another confirmatory inspection. Indeed, all was well. I caught the bus to Odense town hall, where I would change to a second bus for Fruens Bøge. On arriving at the town hall, I was overcome with the feeling that something had been left switched on. There was nothing for it but to wait for a bus to take me the 3 km or so back to university. Sure enough, all was well in the laboratory, just as a more rational bit of my brain seemed to be saying all along. Arriving by bus a second time at the town hall, the same insecurity prevailed. It was now getting late and I was torn as to what to do. A taxi was the only way to have one last look at the laboratory. The driver waited for me while I checked and then drove me to Fruens Bøge. That did finally settle the issue for that day.

What was I afraid of during this checking? What pulled me to do it? I can't say, but using my conscious thoughts as evidence would suggest that it was the need to avoid a catastrophe, such as the university going up in flames. On one level, I knew all was well; on another level, I just doubted it.

Did I remember switching the apparatus off? Maybe. It seemed to me that the essence was in terms of using my memory. On the one hand, intellectually, I knew that the apparatus was switched off. Had

I been asked by a bookie to estimate the chances, I would have given at least 1,000 to 1 in favour. But, on the other hand, I couldn't use that same memory to move on to another activity. It was as if the decision mechanism would scan for problems before allowing me to start a new activity. The memory got corrupted in this decision process.

The fear was that I would be responsible if a disaster were to happen, because I had left something switched on. I thought maybe the switch that I recalled being down was really up. Could it be that my attention had wandered while at the crucial stage in the check? I might remember well enough touching the switch, but perhaps I actually pushed the switch up while pressing it to make 100 per cent sure it was down. Perhaps I was deceiving myself and the memory I was then reviewing was that from yesterday's check rather than today's. One last check will do it, and so on . . . Some investigators believe that the basis of checking is a concern to prevent guilt or criticism.

Apart from wasting time on checking doors and electric switches, I spent time checking the contents of letters. I would write several letters, seal them and take them to the post, only to feel insecure that I had put the right letter in the right envelope. I would then open them up to read their contents. My friend David Booth could never have realised just how many envelopes addressed to him ended up in the rubbish-bin for every one sent.

Where does the motivation for checking come from? For checking gas taps, it could be argued that it is an exaggeration of a perfectly rational fear of a fire. It is difficult to see, though, what awful consequence could follow mixing up letters, at least of the sort I was writing that concerned motivation in rats! I guess that in some cases the obsessional's craving for personal perfection has a lot to do with it. Things have to be exactly right, there must be no room for doubt. One's standing in life might fall if a curious letter were to arrive on the desk of an associate. Like a child, the obsessional craves assurance and comfort, and is locked in a fruitless search for security. Nothing must be left to chance. Even harmless errors must be prevented in the relentless pursuit of perfection. However, in some cases it is difficult to see by any stretch of logic that something bad is being avoided; for example, an obsessional might spend hours checking that books on a shelf are aligned correctly.

For me, things were now going from bad to worse; serious depression was setting in. Depression in the past, present or future is often associated with obsessive compulsive disorders. Some writers characterise the phase of depression following a period of obsessional rumination as being one in which the individual has no more fight left to oppose the obsession. Graham Reed describes this by military analogy as a surrender to the intrusion instead of the previous combat. I certainly felt now that I had exhausted all of the fight that had been in me. I had no intellectual tricks up my sleeve, no new modes of living, no way of looking at the world that was able even to begin to fight hard enough against the curse.

Associated with the depression, my sleep was very badly affected. I awoke early in the morning, unable to get back to sleep (a well-recognised symptom of depression). On the other hand, by day, I was so tired that I had difficulty in concentrating. Several times people came to my office, to find me in an exhausted state, slumped over my typewriter. Something was pulling me downhill fast and there appeared to be no brake. I looked half-dead and it was apparent to all that things were seriously wrong. My associates in the department asked me what was happening.

The world is perceived so differently through the eyes and ears of a depressive. The Danish language, which had brought such a thrilling challenge and later allowed assimilation into a new culture, now sounded unpleasant. It irritated me and was alien, ugly and threatening. I switched to the security of English whenever I could.

I told the psychiatrist of my utter despair. He said that the only solution left was for me to be hospitalised and to receive electroconvulsive therapy. He would, however, be reluctant to prescribe this, because I needed my brain for academic work, and he couldn't rule out memory impairment. I left his office and took a shortcut through the Hans Christian Andersen gardens to get back to the city centre. I had taken a similar route some 20 months earlier, on leaving the restaurant with Winnie. Then I had just arrived in Denmark and was full of enthusiasm for life; now I was a broken man. The memory from 20 months earlier came back and tortured me.

On travelling around Odense, I would look out of the bus window at car drivers and pedestrians and think to myself 'I bet you are well. You are not suffering as I am. Why me? Why not you? You've never had this cross to bear.' By a curious logic, I also felt cheated, because this was all unexpected. So often in England and after arriving in Denmark, I had predicted and planned for potential disasters that would take my new-found paradise away from me. The Danish *Fremskrits* Party might be elected and close Odense University but I had done all in my power to become assimilated into this land. If that were to happen,

Copenhagen University would surely offer something. Nothing could surely go wrong that hadn't been anticipated and ruminated about, but now it had. Like at Singapore in World War II, the guns were all pointing in the wrong direction.

One of the symptoms of depression is a tendency for the person to distort what, by popular consensus, is reality. Among other things, this distortion consists of self-devaluation, sometimes done to a gross extent. Later, and with the benefit of hindsight, I was able to see that I was massively devaluing my abilities and potential. Of course, one gets into a vicious circle, where the devaluation can become a self-fulfilling prophesy. That apart, devaluation can also be applied to things for which there are more objective ways of assessment. By any criterion our study on the computer simulation of feeding was coming along very well. In only four years' time David Booth was to publish an influential book of readings, inspired by our work. Objectively speaking, I just had to get well and I would have interesting challenges. But I couldn't see it that way. To me, the future would be such that, whether healthy or not, there would be nothing more for me to do as a scientist. I felt guilty accepting my salary cheque from the University. I was finished. There were no more avenues of challenge to go down. There were no more books that I could write, because I had nothing more to say. The truth is, and would have been obvious to anyone else, that the potential was enormous. Twenty-seven years and ten books later, I feel that I have only scratched the surface of motivation theory. My professor tried to give me guidance but I was not receptive. I never once doubted my moral worth as an individual. I didn't feel guilty about anything, except my salary cheque. I saw myself unambiguously as a victim and felt no personal responsibility in how I had led my life up till then.

There was now a real danger that Mette, who was voicing fears for her own mental health, would be dragged down with me. She had just got a place at university to read for a law degree. She tried to help for a while but simply could not cope with this nightmare. Her helplessness was total, for what could she possibly do? She felt that everything was right in our relationship, as did I. It was not so long ago that we had discussed buying a new house in Odense. What could we do? Suppose I went into a mental hospital in Denmark. Then I thought of the unthinkable: suppose psychiatric care were better in Britain. Maybe I needed to leave Denmark, return home and find out. Mette and I discussed this endlessly, concluding for no good reason that psychiatric care might be better in the UK.

Could all this really be happening to me? When one feels like a help-less child, is there no one to appeal to, a kind of psychiatric policeman or ombudsman who will somehow sort out one's life? This country seemed so sweet a little while ago. I felt certain that it was now a matter of life and death, and so I got compassionate leave from the University.

The next three days were spent in a state of endless rumination about death, my health and future. Should I leave or should I stay? My mind was made up and then unmade, time after agonising time. Schemes and plans were entertained and then the dread of their implications turned me against them. When things seemed utterly insoluble, thoughts of climbing the highest building in Odense, the hospital, came into my consciousness. No – I couldn't take that way out of it. I ate almost nothing. My weight, already low (well below 64 kg, for a height of 1.83 m), now slipped down still further. Night merged into day, and nightmares were muddled with reality. The only mercy was a period of sleep from about midnight to 3 a.m. Something radical had to be done and at last the strength came to me to make the decision to go.

I sneaked away from University without properly saying goodbye to anyone, not even Mette. It was all too painful, feeling that, for better or worse, I would not be coming back. Mette would only discover that I had gone when she got home and read my desperate note. I would write to Lars, my professor, from England. A taxi took me to Fruens Bøge, I picked up all of my essential worldly possessions, and we were quickly at Odense station. Now there really must be no turning back, even if things were temporarily to get worse.

The boat-train *Englaenderin* had left Copenhagen that morning and now it pulled into Odense. This was the same type of mauve train that had often taken me to the capital, for work or for relaxation at Mette's home, always in pleasure. But now the screech of its brakes evoked no awe in me, no revival of happy memories from childhood train-spot-ting days in Cambridge; that noise like any other now served only to accentuate the terror that I was already feeling. This was the terror of the helpless and hopeless, those who feel they can no longer exert any control over destiny.

A group of carefree Danes were in my compartment laughing and drinking. I found a window seat, and soon we were under way to the port of Esbjerg. A blonde and blue-eyed Scandinavian woman was on the platform waving goodbye to a friend. In one respect, my sexual drive was zero if not actually negative right then, but at another level, almost sadistically, the memories were still intact and their awful tantalising significance was not lost on me. Could I be making a gigantic mistake in leaving? Maybe I had not yet exhausted all the possibilities. Perhaps there existed a new drug, if only I could find the right expert. My eyes followed the marvellous form of the woman on the platform as she, and then the town of Odense, receded into the distance. I asked myself 'How could life be so cruel? How can such beauty exist in the midst of suffering? What might England offer me?'

My family were pleased to welcome me back home in Histon. My father had been worried sick when he knew that I was in trouble, offering to fly out to the rescue. He showed obvious signs of delight at getting me back in one piece. I visited friends in the village and relatives came to see me. I cycled around Cambridgeshire, preoccupied with what to do. I ruminated about future possibilities. Should I go to see the village GP? Have I any useful contacts here? Then in the midst of these ruminations it occurred to me – I was having fewer intrusions about death. Come to think of it, even in the last few days in Denmark, the other problems that I was debating, to stay or go, were causing so much anguish that they pushed death into second place. Things might be bad now, but at least they were less bad and differently bad. Thank God for small mercies, or rather in this case big mercies. I had something to ruminate over that was, at least in principle, within my control.

Should I stay or risk moving away from Histon to return to academia? I applied for a job at Hatfield Polytechnic, which was not too far away, was offered an interview, but declined it out of cowardice. I felt I was not up to it, which, on reflection, was patently nonsensical.

I spent a weekend in Brighton with some friends. Passionate political debate, laughter and a party were good for my spirit. Yes, death was slowly losing some of its potency, but why? Was it simply being usurped by the demands of choosing a future? That weekend in Brighton I wrote my letter of resignation from Odense but couldn't find the courage to post it. What could the future hold for me if I did post it? Unemployment? On returning to Cambridge via London, I stopped for a bite to eat in the Charing Cross Road. A young couple were sitting in the restaurant and my attention was drawn to the attractiveness and style of the woman. I looked at her for as long as would be decent for an Englishman. Then I heard the sound that I wanted least of any in the world to hear: they started speaking Danish. That experience made dropping the resignation letter in the postbox at Leicester Square all the more agonising, but at last I found the courage to do so.

7
Getting back to normal

*'Reader, amidst the difficulties and dangers of this life, should you
ever be tempted to despair, call to mind these latter chapters of the life
of Lavengro. There are few positions, however difficult, from which
dogged resolution and perseverance may not liberate you.'*
GEORGE BORROW, *Lavengro*

A vacancy had arisen in the Psychology Department at Preston
Polytechnic (now University of Central Lancashire). I applied and was
given the date for an interview. Cowardice shortly took over: I declined
the interview. Then I became worried about not finding another job,
so I rang Mike Stone, the head of department, and asked him to negate
my cancellation, which he very kindly did.

The people conducting my interview were a nice group. When they
offered me the post I accepted. I returned to Histon but again got scared
of the unknown, so after some weeks I wrote to Preston to decline the
offer. I then thought that this was an awful mistake. Having to make
a decision was a terrible experience; I tried to put it off as long as possible. I would make a provisional decision, accept it and then search
for disadvantages associated with the choice. I would switch to the
alternative but immediately search the new choice for flaws. As I read
the *Guardian* in bed each morning, I told myself 'just one more page
and you must get up and face it'. I was always able to find a new excuse
to put off making each decision.

Three days after posting my second resignation to Preston, I visited
David Booth in Birmingham, feeling very low. My emotions were combined fear and depression but watching David at work in the University
was a vivid reminder of just how attractive this profession is.

I looked at David's phone and thought 'perhaps the letter has not
arrived yet in Preston. I might pre-empt it. They might still want me.'
David was talking about the motivational significance of the rate at
which food leaves a rat's stomach, a subject having a particular appeal
for him – and me too when times were better. My mind was not with
him: my thoughts were hovering between Preston and Histon. Perhaps

if I were to ring, they will confirm that I no longer have the job and that could resolve it. But the first term's teaching load was not heavy. Surely I could do it. Do I want the job or not? Could David help? Should I seek his advice? No. I must decide.

That afternoon I used David's phone to ring the head of department, quite expecting to be told where to go. Yes, he had received the letter. The computer had been told and had deleted me. He did understand my problem. But could I change my mind one last time? Yes!!

* * *

It started to rain as my train pulled into Wigan. Somehow arriving there in the grey of evening didn't have quite the romantic appeal of seeing Copenhagen in the morning sun, but I was prepared to settle for a life without glamour now. At Preston station, Maurice McCullough, senior lecturer in psychology, was waiting with his dog. He took me to his house where I had been invited to stay, adding 'I wondered whether you would really be on the train!' It was good being with Maurice and his wife Camille, and I was made so welcome. Irish hospitality was just what I needed to complete my recovery. I soon found a flat, in an attractive part of town, overlooking Avenham Park. The students were a friendly and lively bunch and life was good.

I phoned Mette to tell her the good news that stability prevailed and she visited me shortly afterwards. The experience in Preston felt like being snatched from the jaws of death, and in a strange way I was convinced that it would not be necessary to go through such suffering again. Just walking around Preston doing the shopping took on a delight.

Among other things, the department put me in charge of entertainment. A local disco was hired and my flat was used for student parties. Some memorable jokes were told and got passed on to future generations of Preston students. Every day I thought back to Denmark and sighed inwardly at the relief of having escaped from the torture of mental illness.

At Christmas 1974, I met Helen at a party put on by a psychology student. I had earlier ogled her from afar at an election meeting but was not able to talk to her. I liked what she had to say to me and it matched her stunning good looks. We soon formed a partnership.

After about six months in Preston there were just a few signs that all was not going entirely as it should. However, seen in the context of earlier events, it did not amount to a package of symptoms that caused me worry. Nightmares came back. To be precise, they were now more often night terrors. Sometimes the generic term 'nightmare' is used to cover both the true nightmare and the very much rarer and more serious condition of night terror (also termed *pavor nocturnus*) in which the heart rate is massively accelerated because of the terrifying experience. I would wake up screaming in the night or crying out for help. The terror was indescribable. Sometimes I would simply scream and sit up or jump out of bed, never being able to articulate any associated thought process. Usually, I could easily return to sleep afterwards, a somewhat surprising aspect of this condition. Very occasionally, I didn't remember anything about the nocturnal activity, until Helen told me the next day. More commonly the same simple theme would reappear regularly; my breathing was being arrested, or I had poison placed in my mouth and I had to expel it. This would prompt a rush to the bathroom as I desperately tried to rid my mouth of the substance. An attacker might appear and I would leap from the bed to evade his knife. At times the threat was one I would be unable to define, of the kind 'this is it – you are going to die now, this second'. The theme was always a single image corresponding to a single event in the outside world, like one or two frames frozen and cut from a horror movie. Sometimes I would be falling and would awake gaining my balance. The falling theme was particularly likely to occur very soon after passing into sleep. The themes had one important feature in common: they were always ones involving me as the victim; I was never the violent party.

In addition to night terrors, a compulsive checking ritual reappeared. On leaving my flat I would check again and again that the door really was secured. In fact, if anything, this threatened rather than increased my security, since the lock was positively weakened by the strain of testing. I was also cautious about possible disasters ahead, predicting accidents of various kinds, but, in spite of all this, my mood could be described as very happy and 'well', and I was working efficiently.

Paradoxically, I noticed that the intensity of the fear of a disaster declined as the event in question got nearer in time. The intrusive thoughts themselves seemed to be much worse than performing the action that they concerned. For example, a planned journey down the motorway would evoke considerable fear until the day of departure. The journey itself would present little or no problem. Anticipated fear as measured by the frequency of intrusions would be all the greater if there were no unambiguous reason for engaging in the activity. A motorway journey would evoke more anticipatory fear if it were possible to travel to the destination by rail instead. A journey would also present more fear if I had no way out of the commitment. A casual invitation would evoke little fear even if I knew that in all probability I would take it up, provided I could always feel that it was possible to get out of it.

In 1976 I was asked by David McFarland to serve as external DPhil examiner for a candidate at Oxford. Richard Dawkins was the internal examiner. On the way to the Zoology/Psychology building, I purchased a copy of *Breakdown*, an account of a nervous breakdown written by my professor at Sussex, Stuart Sutherland. The *viva voce* was followed that evening by a celebratory party, a wonderful occasion, rich in fun and intellectual stimulation.

David McFarland later escorted me back to his home where I was to spend the weekend. I stayed up late that night reading *Breakdown*, and was distressed to read of Stuart's suffering. So much of it rang true after my experiences. It was rather cold in the bedroom and I kept on a pullover while I was reading. I got up to where Stuart was lying in the street in Naples screaming from mental torment and then I put the book down. I put out the light and dropped off to sleep. Suddenly, in my dream, I was being sucked into a building by my poloneck sweater, which had got caught in the ventilation propeller. I fought to resist, but all I could do was to tear off the collar, let that be sucked in, and thereby try to escape. On awakening the next morning I found to my horror that in reality I had indeed torn the neck off my pullover and it was lying on the bed.

In the following months, the intrusions were still there at low frequency. It was like the days in Denmark before things got bad. However, I felt myself to be master of my fate and captain of my soul. The intrusions at that time were like having a medium-to-bad cold, whereas the latter stages in Denmark had been like a kidney stone. Anyone unfortunate enough to have experienced the latter will know what I mean! I didn't think that I would sink again, but I would rather have been without the intrusions. Life between 1974 and 1978 was good. I still basked in the joy of escaping from permanent mental torment.

8
Misplaced complacency

'He may even believe, at an unconscious level, that he can avoid death altogether, if only he gives the problem enough time, thought and effort.'

Dr Allan Mallinger,
The Obsessive's Myth of Control

In 1978 I got a job at the Open University, and Helen and I moved down to Milton Keynes in September. At the stage where I was getting used to the Open University, the intrusions were still there but at a relatively low frequency and intensity, still like a cold rather than a kidney stone. However, after five years of being in Milton Keynes, I felt that it might be worth seeing whether British medicine and psychiatry had anything to offer.

I felt odd talking to my GP about this, wishing that I had come with a 'proper illness', like tonsillitis or an ingrowing toenail. He gave me a sympathetic hearing, saying 'This fascinates me. I wish I had time to devote myself to it. I sometimes look at the stars at night, and wonder what it's all about. It's occasionally uncomfortable.' He referred me to a local clinical psychologist.

The clinical psychologist tried two techniques to counter the intrusive thoughts. One consisted of getting me to place a rubber band around my wrist, and to ping it whenever an unwanted thought intruded. At the same time I was to give myself a silent message of the kind 'Go away' or 'You are not wanted'. If I were able to anticipate the intrusion by getting in with the ping first, so much the better. That is to say, I should try to identify the cues that trigger the thought and react to them with corrective action. To this end, it was necessary to record a sample of situations in which intrusions occurred. I found this no easy task. Imagine how easy it is to disturb a psychological process by monitoring it, particularly when the observer and the observed are one and the same concerned individual. There are few better stimuli to ruminate than a notebook of ruminations but therapists are well aware of this problem.

The observations were started while I was on a visit to Holland and West Germany; time, content of the thought, intensity (on a scale from 0 to 8, the worst possible) and duration were recorded. Typical observations were:

- arrival in Hagen → feeling: how nice to be here → nice now, but will not last (intensity 5, duration 10 minutes),

- at breakfast a waiter congratulates me on my German → good feeling → my forthcoming stay here → but it can't last (intensity 3, duration 5 minutes),

- train passes cemetery → my own death (intensity 4, duration 5 minutes),

- two Turkish *Gastarbeiter* ('guest workers') pass me in the street → immigration → recent neo-Nazi activity → a recent arson attack on some Turks → my own death (intensity 2, duration 10 minutes).

A pattern was emerging. As an approximation, I could divide the intrusions into three classes:

1. those triggered by a positive cue, such as receiving congratulations, reflecting upon good in the future or being reminded of one's worth,

2. those triggered by a negative cue, such as reading about a plane crash or an obituary or being reminded of the passage of time,

3. no obvious cue present, 'spontaneous intrusions'.

Consider where the waiter told me that I speak good German – 'Hoch Deutsch'. This was an example of type 1, something to make one feel good. Contrast this with passing a cemetery, a typical type 2, a rather obvious one linked to the morbid. Somewhat more subtle, but still in class 2, is someone saying 'it's your birthday next month', and thereby reminding me of the passage of time. The division was roughly one-third falling into each of the three categories.

There was also a time factor involved. The time most free of intrusions was upon waking, particularly if I could afford the luxury of lying in bed for a while with no particular immediate purpose. Paradoxically, at other times, the best situation would be one of hard work in which there was little or no scope for free-flowing thoughts.

The thoughts invariably concerned either the future in its own right or the past as an index of the passage of time: 'The last year seemed to fly past' or 'It can't be a year since then'. Thus ruminations were never over past events themselves or how the past might have been. Even nostalgia for the past, for the music of the sixties or for my schooldays, did not have a negatively toned quality to it. Such thoughts have always been pleasant.

The technique of thought-stopping seemed not to work. I then attempted to convert thought-stopping into a schedule of punishment. In response to an intruding thought, I would pull the elastic band rather far and then let it go, which certainly felt like punishment. I would also pinch my skin hard for the thought to be really punished, but this didn't seem to work either.

Back in Milton Keynes the clinical psychologist was very interested in these results and tried a second technique. He invited me to think about a morbid theme, to deliberately trigger the intrusion. Then, having told me to close my eyes, he would slam a book down on the table, shouting 'STOP', I think that the STOP instruction might have had some slight effect but it was weak at best.

On my own initiative I then tried visiting a hypnotist in London. He produced a tape of the session, which contained the following messages among others.

'You are going now into a peaceful and calm world. There is nothing to bother you. Now relax. It is a beautiful day and you are lying on a sandy warm beach.

'Looking back on the time when you used to be anxious you can now put that out of your mind. Now see yourself as the person you want to be. Not allowing pessimism and worry to dog you.'

Unlike in Denmark, this time I was very receptive to hypnotism. I also tried the Alexander technique, being taught by Alexander's nephew, which certainly helped my posture, if not my mind! I suffered no more backaches. His first question to me was 'Have you ever been in the army?'

'No, why?'

'Because your posture is so stiff, as if you were on a parade ground. Try to lower your shoulders. You don't need to clench your fists!'

Yoga, which I tried at about the same time, had an immediate and dramatic effect on reducing the frequency and intensity of ruminations but the effect was short-lived. I think that there remained a residual small benefit from regular practice. Hard physical exercise, jogging and particularly aerobics had a good effect, as did listening to the hypnosis tape. It seemed that there was no magic cure but I could hold the enemy at bay with passive resistance or 'hand-to-hand fighting'.

Helen and I took a holiday in Ireland, visiting Londonderry briefly. Later, in Eire, we stared hard at the statue of the Virgin Mary in Ballinspittle, Co. Cork, which was said to move. It failed to do so for us but the visit was fascinating. One day we were wandering around Dublin, and Helen remarked: 'I think that it was here last year where the coach driver told us not to walk around. It's a tough part of town.'

We didn't think too much about this; after all, unlike in New York, the people in Ireland looked just like us. A few seconds later someone pounced and grabbed me round the neck from behind. I immediately thought of Canice, an Irish student at Preston. At a flash, in my mind, he had spotted his former tutor and wanted to surprise us. Obsessionals can sometimes be hopelessly naïve optimists! Being somewhat less of a naïve optimist, Helen quickly let out a piercing scream and I felt a hand tugging violently at my money. No, it wasn't Canice. On failing to destabilise me and get my money, he fled.

In 1984 and 1985, I spent two periods abroad, at the Ruhr University in Bochum, West Germany, and Claude Bernard University in Lyon, France. Each of these visits was a spectacular success and I loved my time there. On my first Saturday in Bochum I took the tram down to the market to do the week's shopping and felt once again that warm glow of my first year in Odense. I had great fun in the town's bars, and memories of an evening spent at *Trauminsel* will be with me forever.

The next year in France the sun also shone brightly on my life, and the food was better than in Germany. By request, in the lunch hours I taught conversational English informally to the staff who needed it – secretaries, technicians and even the occasional academic. I was often invited to their homes for meals, the wine was good and flowed freely; this was truly a great period in my life. I would sometimes take the high-speed train (*Le TGV*) to Paris at the weekend, and get a thrill out of the big-city life. I felt the cares of the world disappear in the bustle of the Metro, with the help of an earlier glass or two of wine. The smell of the Metro always evokes a wonderful emotion in me.

The ruminations were at a relatively low level in France but I was curious to see whether anything might be available to help. One day I was having an intimate tête-à-tête with Jacques Mouret in Lyon, and he described his electrical brain stimulation technique for helping depressives and heroin addicts. I went to the hospital on several occasions, and had current passed through my brain for an hour or so. Whether it changed the state of my central nervous system, I am not sure, but certainly the sight of the nurse in charge of the apparatus did.

Back in Britain, I missed Lyon very much, but managed to readapt to Milton Keynes.

9
Never get complacent

*'And as time went on the thought of death began to haunt him till
it became a constant obsession. In the daytime, fascinated by it,
he would lay down his pen and sit brooding on it; at night, he would
lie tossing feverishly from side to side, with the blackness that was
awaiting ever before him. And with the sickly light of the early
morning, there met him the early relief of having dragged on
one day nearer the end.*

'A conflict of egoisms' in *Wreckage*
by HUBERT CRACKANTHORPE, 1893

The thoughts were still at a low frequency. However, trying to eliminate them, I wrote to Professor Jeffrey Gray, at the Institute of
Psychiatry in London, whom I had met on a couple of occasions. I was
in the process of writing a book for a series of which he was general
editor. His predecessor as professor of psychology, Hans Eysenck, had
pioneered behaviour therapy (exposure to the feared situation) for
phobias and compulsive behaviour. I would have taken this course of
action much earlier had my problem been essentially behavioural.
Jeffrey suggested that I contact an associate of his, Padmal de Silva. By
coincidence, I had just read an article by him, comparing Buddhist and
behaviourist techniques of controlling unwanted thoughts.

Padmal talked at length to me and was most sympathetic. I liked
him immediately. He suggested that I write out the content of the
intrusions and record them on tape; I should then play them back to
myself. When patients are told that treatment consists of exposure
to the very stimulus that they most dread, they sometimes decline it
out of fear. However, this technique appealed to me; it fitted my
preference for methods close to behaviourist psychology. The logic
behind it is simple: if something is repeated enough times with no
significant consequence, it tends to lose its attention value. The
ticking of a clock is an obvious example. In my case, I would flood
myself with intrusions in the hope to *habituate* them – that, ideally,
they would thereby fade into 'nothing'.

Padmal admitted that nothing in this area is certain: the technique works for some people but not others. As a psychologist, I was in a good position to appreciate this. I should come back in three weeks' time to report progress. Padmal then announced that we were both invited to Hans Eysenck's 70th birthday party. It was a jolly and pleasant occasion. The lively conversation made me realise that I still had my sense of humour, in spite of the ordeal before me, and I left as always in an optimistic mood. Such optimism in a treatment might be expected to have the effect, if any, of increasing its success, the so-called 'placebo effect'. Also, it is often argued that a trusting rapport with the therapist is a major factor in the success of any therapy. Padmal gave me some scientific papers to read, suggested I get hold of *Living with Fear* by Isaac Marks and wished me well. These papers were to lead ultimately to this book.

I employed free association (letting the mind run freely from one item to another, with no conscious steering) to generate as many intrusions as possible. It was not difficult to fill a few sides of A4. My recording, involving names of psychologists most meaningful to me, went like this:

> 'J Watson is dead. Edward Tolman is dead. Like them, you too will one day be dead. There is nothing that you can do to avoid it. Try as hard as you like, it will catch you. Who knows when? Ten years, 20 years, 50 years? One thing is certain; it will find you wherever you may try to hide. Who knows how you will die? You can't say. What will happen to your body after death? No one can say. Only one thing is certain: it will find you and everyone close to you. Your father and sister will go just like you.'

I guess that this sample is enough to give you a feel for the general theme! I made a 20-minute tape like that, and played it with the same enthusiasm that I had had earlier for learning foreign languages. Shaving, eating and dressing were accompanied by this macabre message, rather than a day's conversation in the life of a Danish or Yugoslavian family.

Much to my regret both as client and psychologist, after three weeks I was unable to report any success. I discussed this at length with Padmal, and he suggested a variation on the theme. Rather than develop the full richness of the thoughts, it might be better to record one single thought: 'You will die'. I should put aside up to two hours each day just listening to this message. I should not try to economise on time by shaving or eating while the tape was playing, it needed to be my sole concern. Furthermore, it would be better to listen to the message through earphones, by means of which it would seem to originate in my head. After some thousands of exposures, any decrease could be compared with a thought that had not been habituated (the 'control condition') – for example, the death of someone close to me. He expressed sympathy and understanding at the prospect of a not very pleasant experiment. Again though, after trying this technique, I felt no diminution in the power of the thought to evoke a negative reaction. Death was as bad at the end of each session as at the beginning, and I could perceive no decline between sessions.

I then 'invented' a technique that was a variation on an experiment of Pavlov's and used since in behavioural therapy. Pavlov had shown that if an unpleasant event is immediately followed by a pleasant one, the unpleasant one sometimes loses its negative effect and can even seem to acquire a positive aspect. For example, a dog will even come to salivate rather than jump when given a mild electric shock, if the shock heralds food. So how could an unpleasant intrusion be followed by something positive? A pleasant thought – sex? I discussed this with Padmal. We both realised that there is a danger that, rather than death becoming less negative, one might become frightened by sex. What would be a pleasant thought, but one not quite so fundamental? We arrived at Indonesian food. Even if I were to develop an aversion to this, though unfortunate for my visits to Holland, it would not be catastrophic; I could always eat Indian food. To every morbid thought, I answered with thoughts of a plate of *gado gado* or *tahu goreng*. It seemed not to work but was worth the try.

Padmal questioned me closely on the exact nature of the intruding thoughts, with a view to gaining control over them. What sensory form did they take – did I experience, say, simply a kind of visual image in my mind in which I 'saw' something related to death? Instead, or in addition to this, was the obsessional theme represented in terms of a series of thoughts with meanings and implications ('semantically')? In other words, was it as if I were speaking death-related ideas and puzzles to myself?

A fundamental aspect of humans (as well as other animals) is our desire to have control over a situation. Take control away and something vital is lost. Trying to gain some control over even intrusive thoughts might lower their intensity. For example, suppose someone's intrusive thought is always of a coffin in a particular position. The person can try to turn this image in her mind, or change its distance from her as observer. I tried to recall the exact form that the intrusions took but this was surprisingly difficult. I had not been required before to consider the problem in this way – I had just lived with it on and off for 13 years. My recollection was that, in general, there was no one single image or form. The exact content varied. For periods of a month or so, a distinct visual form would tend to dominate. I would see myself in a coffin in church. That would be followed the next month by seeing myself six feet underground. Sometimes I would visualise the flames of the crematorium. At other times, death would take a more abstract form. I would see (yes, I think 'see' is right) a dimension marker like those used by draughtsmen extending from now to about 40 years into the future, with a clear end-point indicated. The marker would nudge me with 'It's limited, it will not last forever'.

At times the intrusions were abstract, almost cryptic. A joyful anticipation would trigger it – 'it' being, as best I can describe it, a feeling of 'negative emotion' that had no immediate sensory thought content. 'It' was almost independent of the death thought – we might imagine this feeling as serving as a messenger that all is not well. Unity was not there. Anticipation was a risky business, because the good would be tainted with the bad. If I were to probe what was going on, to ask myself immediately after feeling the wave of negative emotion what it was about, the associated thought content was clear enough: death.

After extensive discussion with Padmal concerning the richness of content of my intrusions, represented in both visual and semantic forms, we felt that they did not lend themselves to the approach of trying to gain control over the exact form of their content.

The methods of behavioural psychology not having worked, I turned again to my GP for help, suggesting medication. Knowing me to be a psychologist, he asked what I thought. I said that anxiety was the most obvious feature; any depression was secondary to anxiety. Therefore, it would suggest anti-anxiety agents. The choice was between anti-anxiety or anti-depressant tablets, though the distinction is not always a clear one. We settled for anti-anxiety agents, though he wasn't entirely convinced that this was right. These tablets did not seem to help. I then tried beta-blockers – a type of drug that reduces the activity of the heart and thereby reduces the feedback signals to the brain from the heart – but they didn't help either (they were an unusual choice of drug and one that would not generally be recommended for this condition).

In 1986 the ruminations were getting worse again and they were taking a somewhat different character, towards the philosophical. Hitherto their intellectual content had hardly been profound, consisting of repetitions of a few uncomplicated dark thoughts. Now I was being tormented by associated existential dilemmas and theological ideas that might have been fascinating had I been strong enough to take them. But they were bringing me much bother for very little insight; I simply wanted to be rid of them.

Until then, on being asked if I were a Christian, I would reply rather light-heartedly 'If I wake up one day in heaven, I'll believe. Until then I am a card-carrying agnostic.' The question didn't really trouble me, though it was a matter of some detached intellectual fascination. The fear of death was certainly not a fear of divine retribution or theological uncertainty, but simply one of losing my earthly identity. Now the thoughts concerned the insignificance of a mortal existence. This moved me to read a great deal to try to come to terms with the problem. The behavioural scientist Donald Mackay's views on the after-life, the physicist Russell Stannard's on the relation between science and religion, and the work *The Intelligent Universe* by Sir Fred Hoyle, among many others, provided a rich source of stimulation but no answers to reduce the discomfort. Helen and I parted under the strain.

Nothing seemed to add up; it just wouldn't work any way. Being raised on a belief in Darwinian evolution, it was difficult to see why or how a system should need to go through the tortuous stages of evolution to get to us, if it were in some meaningful sense instigated by an omniscient and omnipotent source. On the other hand, purpose is an intrinsic feature of how biological systems work, and so by logical extension one might feel it necessary to impute a purposive quality to the whole evolutionary process. Could God be the end-point rather than the start? The discussions I was hearing from my associates in physics, with time running backwards and subatomic particles seeming to exist for a microsecond only in the eye of the beholder, would permit almost anything to be believed.

To ask how long the physical universe has existed used to be described as being philosophically naïve. Now such a question was again respectable. I ruminated endlessly on these issues, torturing myself with them. The possibility of, the hope of, life after death assumed an inordinate significance for someone who previously would have described the issue as naïve and a waste of time. The distinguished behavioural neuroscientist Professor Donald Mackay made the prospect of a transformation from a physical body to a non-physical one sound almost easy, by comparison with a translation of computer software from one computer to another, but this helped not at all. Indeed, it only fuelled further pointless speculation. Suppose the transformation to the after-life went wrong; by analogy with my experience of computers, an unexpected bug in the translation program could cause havoc. Suppose the transformation yielded only a pale imitation of a conscious being? Suppose there is something about the real biological nerve cells, flesh and blood that yields consciousness, something that could not be captured by a computer program? Suppose? Suppose? Suppose . . . ? Just let me get out of this madhouse!

Hard-nosed mechanistic science (the kind of science that looks for mechanical ('physical') cause-and-effect explanations for everything, including even the mind and spiritual experience) and analogies between humans and rats, in which I had placed so much faith, were now just another source of fear. Something essential was missing, if not in any rational or scientific sense then certainly as far as my psychological needs were concerned. Was I craving the impossible? But this was a real need, a need for security that my science could not provide.

Now the obsessions were accurately characterised not so much as an image or a spoken word, but as a series of related intellectual puzzles, ones that I wanted to be rid of. Life after death triggered the speculation 'why couldn't the world be a secure place where death never intruded?' How could anyone be expected to cope with the vagaries of mortal existence? If only things had been different in the beginning, we might have had an immortal consciousness. If only . . . If only . . . The philosophical dilemma of it all, or 'pathological dilemma' if one prefers the expression, tortured me. It was as if I had been programmed to search out the incongruous, the fearful in everything that impinged on me. The world can be a terrifying place if viewed through such a mental processor, and this one seemed brilliant at finding anxiety- and depression-evoking dilemmas.

I understand how the obsessional, John Bunyan, felt:

'But yet all the things of God were kept out of my sight, and still the tempter followed me with, "But whither must you go when you die? what will become of you? where will you be found in another world? what evidence have you for heaven and glory, and an inheritance among them that are sanctified?" Thus was I tossed for manie weeks, and knew not what to do . . .'

Doubtless Woody Allen could have put some of the content of my more absurd thoughts to productive artistic use, but I could see no humour in any of it.

When the intrusive thought did have a clear visual character, this was now most often of Earth spinning on somewhere in the vast expanse of the universe. How little and insignificant we seemed in all this space. How terrifying was the lack of control over fate implied by this image.

Fear alternated with frustration and jealousy, a kind of egotism and narcissism that one would be ashamed to make public. I didn't even want to contemplate the universe going on without me. I wanted to be 'where it is all at'; I couldn't possibly delegate this to anyone else. No; posterity earned through writing books didn't even begin to answer the need. The possibility of some form of survival in the consciousness of my friends and students was just a mockery of my basic need; there was only one variety of posterity that mattered, the survival of personal consciousness. All else was nonsense. Nothing seemed to be of any value, because nothing would be permanent. Why bother to achieve anything? Every task before me seemed meaningless because none of them would survive. Every goal was measured against the potential mortality of the end-point, and every task of course failed the test.

A paradox was becoming more and more evident. As bad as the intrusive thoughts were, and as strenuous and unambiguous as my efforts to fight them were, when I reflected on the possibility of life without them, this prospect held its own peculiar anxiety. Imagine facing death unexpectedly. At least the way things are at present, it can never catch you unawares. I might even resolve the issue, provided I worked hard enough at it. But if I don't reflect on the issue, there is no chance of resolving it. Could there be a bizarre mechanism at work that was sustaining these thoughts because on one level they were a protection mechanism? Maybe, but what did that lead to? Never for a moment in my actions did I detract from the battle to eliminate the enemy. In November 1986 my mental state moved worryingly downwards. I noticed that my 'startle reaction', always sensitive, was now hyper-sensitive. I walked into my office one day, expecting to find no one there, and was met by my secretary. My reaction was one of intense fear. Things that went even mildly bang in the night put me into a state of immediate panic. My fear level as indexed by the pounding of my heart was sensitive to such normally innocuous sounds as the refrigerator going on and off in a distant room.

The anxiety was bad but perhaps depression was now the most dominant emotion. Feeling desperate, I looked into the possibility of private medical care but was advised against it. I lost both my appetite and my interest for work, and started waking each morning at about 4 a.m. Getting up was a great struggle. I couldn't face the day and I kept telling myself that, if only I could have stayed in bed, things might have been better. Sleeping pills were prescribed for me. I was told to take no more than two in a week, in order to prevent dependence. I stretched it to three. At first, those two or three nights were a great relief, but even the pills could not spare me from the ruminations. The most trivial of tasks seemed utterly daunting; I would find reasons to put off composing even a 'thank you' letter, because I couldn't face the effort involved in writing it.

People looked unattractive to me, and yet paradoxically they all looked so well-adjusted and successful. Their behaviour annoyed me and evoked covert hostility and impatience. Whether shopping or waiting for a bus, the crowd had one thing in common: they were in my way. Then, in a queue, experiencing such a feeling, I might feel guilty when an old lady would turn to me and say 'Sorry I'm slow'. This was a useful reminder that so much of what we perceive depends on our own interpretation. In spite of my intolerance, I was frightened to be alone. I tried to engineer the week ahead to make sure that I always had someone around me. People at work said that I looked ill.

A few weeks before this decline I had obtained a new book on obsessions, *Obsessional Experience and Compulsive Behaviour – a Cognitive-structural Approach* by Professor Graham Reed, and read it with interest. Reed argued for antidepressants as a treatment for obsessions. Knowing that British GPs do not always appreciate being told by their patients what to prescribe, it was with some reservation that I took Reed's book with me to the next appointment. However, my own GP has a rather progressive approach and has said that he always appreciated having an 'expert witness' as patient. He agreed that it would be wise to try antidepressants, and prescribed flupentixol (Fluanxol) for me. Unfortunately, it had little desirable effect, and induced tiredness and an inability to concentrate, a zombie-like state.

I visited some GP friends of mine, Barbara and Richard, in Coventry, and they recommended the powerful antidepressant clomipramine (Anafranil). The next day I had an appointment with a local psychiatrist and I mentioned their advice. He too felt that this would be a wise choice and prescribed it. I told him that I might be sinking but at least

I will go down with a fight. 'That's the spirit. Fight it,' he replied. 'You won't sink.'

A low dosage of 10 mg of Anafranil per day was to be increased progressively to 75 mg per day. These tablets seemed to work well for me. My appetite came back. Healthy workaholic tendencies re-emerged and sleep was much improved. The intrusions were less frequent and certainly less frightening. I was back in control again. The only undesirable side-effects were the relatively minor ones of mid-day tiredness, excessive yawning at times and a dry mouth, particularly in the morning. Some of these problems can be answered to some extent by taking a glass of water to bed with you and trying to steal a 10-minute nap at lunchtime. I put on a significant and unwelcome amount of weight.

Both the psychiatrist and my GP were very pleased with the results but the psychiatrist said he saw Anafranil as being only a kind of first aid. In the longer term, the answer would probably lie in some form of psychotherapy. I have the usual behaviourist suspicion of psycho-analysis but do not feel so antagonistic towards other forms of therapy. The psychiatrist announced that a clinical psychologist, Hilary Edwards, trained in cognitive therapy, had just joined the Milton Keynes practice and recommended that I see her.

An example of part of our conversation went something like this.

'What bothers you about death? Is it a fear of what might happen to you after death or a fear of the process of dying?'

'Well ... er ... it is a fear, true, but sometimes perhaps not so much a fear as such but more a disappointment, a frustration, it messes things up to know that they won't last ... it is a fear and a regret in one ... er ... it's difficult to explain really.'

'Yes, I know that it is difficult, but are you saying that things that must end are intrinsically of little value? Do only eternal things have value?'

'Yes ... I guess so, ... sort of ...'

'Have you ever had a really good holiday?'

'Yes.'

'But that had to end. Because it had to end, and you knew that it had to end, did that make it not valuable?'

'No ...'

In this way, the therapist tries to give the client some tools to recon-struct the way he or she sees the world. It is more subtle than pinging elastic bands or repeated exposure. It tries to reshape thought processes that have become automatic and self-reinforcing.

The cognitive therapist invited me to try to find some constructive answers to the obsessional thoughts. For example, in response to the intrusion 'death will come', one might find that its impact can be neutralised to some extent by thinking 'Yes, it will, but that is something beyond my power to worry about. I must concentrate on what I can do at this moment, and leave such matters to others. It will probably be all right on the night.' I tried that counter-cognition repeatedly but I didn't manage to convince myself. The technique did not work for me.

In response to 'all will end' one might try 'We can't be sure that all will end. We simply don't know what will happen. Let's wait and see.'

Another technique that we tried was role reversal. The therapist argues for the motion, in this case that death is something to fear and dread, and the client attempts to marshal arguments against it. The exchange went something like this:

'It's just not worth it. I might as well die.'

'But surely it is worth it. Your husband and child need you.'

'But as it will end, it all makes no sense now to bother about anything. I really couldn't care less about life unless it is eternal life.'

'But you don't act that way. Your actions are those of someone who does value even a mortal existence . . .'

This is something that you can try out with a partner or friend.

But does any of this work? I don't think it helped me much to explore my thoughts but it might help some people. I concluded that there is no magic solution. Each of these techniques can possibly help in a little way to undermine the power of the intrusions.

I had now established a correspondence with Graham Reed, in which we exchanged ideas about intrusive thoughts. Professor Reed urged me to go public, arguing that I would have a valuable contribution to make. I resisted but soon saw the wisdom of putting my thoughts together.

Clomipramine having rescued me, life proceeded smoothly and got better. The intrusions were still there, but at a low frequency and intensity and I felt resigned to them. I could live with them. A person might have a wooden leg and wish that they had one made of flesh and bone, but they can live life nearly to the full. That was how I felt.

Padmal had earlier directed me to the book *Living with Fear* by Isaac Marks. After reading this excellent work, I decided to try a slightly different technique of confronting the intrusions. It is one also described by Viktor Frankl, as 'paradoxical intention'. Rather than lengthy sessions of saturation bombing with thoughts of the kind 'it will happen, it's hopeless', I specifically answered each intrusive thought with a silent thought that was even more negative than the intrusion. Only in response to an unwanted mental event did I present myself with this counter-thought. I confronted myself in my imagination with the worst possible situation that could prevail. For example 'death will come,' I answered with 'of course it will and it will be terrible when it does'. I felt that this worked better than sessions of exposure that were conducted regardless of ongoing mental activity. For me, paradoxical intention was effective.

Now a big event was looming; in June 1987, I was to give the opening talk at an international symposium in Italy on emotion, and I devoted myself to this task. I needed to do a lot of prior reading.

I travelled by train to Pisa. The conference was a wonderful success but during the week my thoughts turned to transport for getting back to England. The journey out by train had been fine, allowing me to visit Paris. But I needed to get back to England soon after the conference. I hadn't flown for 16 years since coming back from Ljubljana, when I was terrified. In the meantime I had been forced to decline invitations to give lectures in, among other places, Moscow and Atlanta. Now was my chance to attempt overcoming the fear. I could try flying on impulse and thereby relatively little anticipation need be involved. Just go to the airport and try to get on the next flight to England.

One of the benefits of being at such a conference is that among the delegates are some of the leading figures on the subject of emotion, with little else to do in the evenings but to drink wine and talk about emotion. I approached Professor Albert Bandura of Stanford University, who emphasised the vital role of trying to gain mastery in any situation of fear. But how at this late stage does one get to master an aircraft, unless you happen to be the pilot? It seemed, though, that I had some minimal potential mastery. I had to go to the airport and buy my ticket. Even at that late stage, I could always opt out and go by train. I could learn something about aircraft. I could try talking to the cabin staff. The wisdom of drinking alcohol was mentioned by my associates, though I guess that one does not need to be a psychologist to know that.

On the Saturday morning, a small group of us, including Vernon Hamilton, a noted expert on obsessionality, and David Warburton, set out by minibus for Pisa airport. The driver fitted exactly one's image of Latins as he negotiated the bends in the road. At this stage, in their extreme discomfort on the back seat, Vernon Hamilton and his wife Betty tried some 'cognitive psychotherapy' on me, to the amusement of the other passengers.

'Are you afraid right now?'

'No. Or rather any fear I might feel is being attributed to the prospect of flying.'

'Good, because you should really be frightened of this journey. Flying will be safer and more comfortable than being in this minibus.'

'Yes. I understand all that, but it isn't really a question of statistics.'

'What are you scared of then?'

'Dying. It's all a question of mastery. I feel that I can influence this driver in some strange way.'

On arriving in one piece at Pisa airport, I proceeded to buy a ticket for London. David Warburton used his knowledge of psychopharmacology to devise a schedule of taking wine. The logic was simple: the alcohol level in my blood should rise most sharply as we boarded the aircraft. David confessed that even as an inveterate traveller he had his fears. 'Alcohol and mastery are the solution; organise your environment when you get on the plane,' he said. 'Ask for a newspaper and a bloody Mary. Have the cabin staff running around you. This will create the feeling that you are master of what goes on.' He then gave me still more the impression of mastery by describing the layout of Pisa airport, the wind direction, the hills that had to be cleared by the aircraft. We observed pilots doing checks of their wing flaps and watched take-offs and landings. It helped to see the faces of pilots. All this made it seem human.

I felt that I could perceive the alcohol soaking into my brain as our flight was called. My emotion was now one of positive excitement rather than fear. As I looked out of the aircraft window, the wave and thumbs-up sign from the ground staff to the pilot was very comforting. It is something I shall never forget. I felt some anxiety as the plane accelerated down the runway but soon the alcohol soothed such lingering doubts. On hearing that I hadn't flown for 16 years, Captain Godfrey asked me into the cockpit and explained the controls. This was just fantastic; I loved it. On arriving at London, I realised I had totally conquered my fear – a testimony to simple exposure as therapy. Now there would be no stopping me; I had 16 lost years to make up.

I had always wanted to visit the Orient – Japan, China or Thailand – but fear of flying had made this impossible. Now, on earning my wings, I immediately consolidated the gain by booking a flight to Bangkok, to take a much-needed holiday in November. I borrowed the Linguaphone 'Teach Yourself Thai' course from the library. By November, I had 'mastered' enough to feel confident with some very small small-talk.

I was able to consume surreptitiously a can of wine before take-off at Heathrow. It was in a calm mood that I boarded the 747 and took into my hand the good-luck charm that a friend had given me for the journey. Take-off was fearless, even exhilarating, as was the rest of the 12-hour journey. Conversation with other passengers was aided by British Airways' regular supply of food and drink. Stepping out of the temperature-controlled plane at Bangkok airport really was like opening an oven door, and the 'Land of smiles' soon lived up to its name. I fought off successive waves of touts and took a bus for Bangkok city. Its traffic had been described to me but the reality surpassed any description. The crazy driving, the heat, the noise, the choking pollution, a particularly obnoxious strain of mosquito – I wondered what the people have got to be so cheerful about, but perhaps such speculation is naïve. The effect is infectious; even the European tourists start smiling at each other.

I travelled a bit around the country and visited a remote settlement of huts where the locals made me welcome. My few Thai expressions came in useful. When they were combined with some English, sign language and drawings, we understood each other reasonably well. I regretted that I had not learned to speak more Thai. After leaving the settlement by a dirt track, I started walking down a road, not knowing where I was heading. Two youths on a motorbike passed, looked at me and stopped. I was greeted with the standard question that Thais love to ask of anyone looking at all foreign:

'Where you go?'
'I go to the town.'
'It's a long way. If you buy me some petrol, I'll take you.'
'How about your companion?'
'He can wait here till I come back for him!'

As we set off dodging the holes in the road and swerving round bends, I suddenly remembered the promise I had faithfully made to my friend in England who gave me the good-luck charm – that I would at all times take care. We arrived safely at our destination and I gave the young man some money for petrol.

Obsessional thoughts were at a very low frequency and intensity. I speculated that the familiar environmental trigger-cues with which they had been associated over the years were mainly absent here; in Bangkok there was little to prime them. One day I experienced the thought sequence (1) Caucasian male approaching, (2) looks like Bertrand Russell, (3) Russell is dead and (4) the inevitability of death. This stood out as being a rare occurrence of an obsessional thought. Whatever the explanation, Thailand was heavenly and free of distractions, at least of the unwanted sort!

It was with a lump in my throat that I boarded the 747 for London. I took no alcohol but felt no fear. Could the emotion of sorrow at leaving new-found friends be inhibiting expression of fear? For whatever reason, I felt sure I had completely cured my fear of flying. I watched the lights of Bangkok receding below as we headed west.

Looking at my behaviour in learning Thai also demonstrated clearly that I was, as always, obsessed with efficiency. Washing up or shaving did not represent an efficient use of time if the mental machinery were lying idle. Learning the rudiments of Thai by the cassettes and shaving was an efficient use of time. Time was treated as a commodity like money or petrol. I was trying to maximise my efficiency, as one might do with a racehorse.

I was, though, enjoying learning Thai very much, and I couldn't wait to get back onto the 747. This year, 1987, had been a good year. City University had awarded me a Doctor of Science for my contribution to psychology. I had no more night terrors, and, thanks to clomipramine, unwanted thoughts were under control. Next year, 1988, looked like being even better.

10
Going public

'This day it came into my mind to write the history of my melancholy. On this I purpose to deliberate; I know not whether it may not too much disturb me.'

SAMUEL JOHNSON

In 1989, my father died aged 89. At once, I lost not only my father but my greatest admirer and one of my best friends as well. Grumpy he might at times have been and bigoted he certainly became, but we didn't want to lose him. Given the availability of word processing then, I had planned to produce for him a copy of this book in large print because his sight was not too good. This would have the added bonus of my being able to remove such slight references to sex as were included, as this was not a topic for a rather puritan household. Alas, such plans were all too late.

The death of course came as a shock but even death can occasionally have a funny side and the funeral bordered on farce at one point. The hearse arrived at the church exactly to plan but, alas, the vicar didn't and we had to launch a search-party for him. To our immense relief, he did appear after a while. My sister found this all very stressful and I was tense but I am ashamed to confess that even then I saw an element of humour in it, as I am sure my father would have. In the service, the vicar mentioned my father's membership of the Home Guard ('Dad's Army') and his great sense of humour (a 'village character'), the irony not being lost on me. At the end of the ceremony, my father's brother Fred remarked to the driver of the hearse, 'Thanks a lot mate – next time you meet me I'll be the one lying out there behind you.'

So, in 1990, the first edition of this book appeared and with it I went public about my psychiatric illness. The book received a large amount of publicity, including a number of appearances on TV (e.g. the ITN national news and *Kilroy*) and radio (e.g. *Woman's Hour*) and reviews in the national and local press.

Some of the reactions were quite predictable but others much less so. One psychologist, a good friend, virtually accused me of imagining things: there was nothing wrong with me, as was perfectly evident from my behaviour. In this regard, I guess that I had myself partly to blame, because the type of psychology that I practise places an emphasis on the behaviour that can be observed rather than the hidden contents of the mind. One article claimed, as far as I could see without a shred of evidence, that I had been a victim of Satanic ritual abuse – and that claim came from one of Britain's most distinguished universities! It is perhaps no wonder that psychologists do not enjoy universal respect.

Many people asked whether writing the book had had a beneficial effect on my own health – a way of getting things out of the system. This kind of logic is very common and obviously taps into an intuitively appealing way of viewing how the brain operates. I cannot say that it did change anything very much and I would not necessarily expect it to do so. If anything, I guess that it served to fuel black thoughts.

A large number of people congratulated me on my courage in going public, which perhaps says something about the stigma of psychiatric illness. In fact, I cannot say that I have ever experienced anything that could be called prejudice, which might indicate something about the relatively open and liberal atmosphere and goals of academia. A politician or army officer might not have been so lucky. However, I soon learned that one of my basic and confident expectations was to be violated: people at the highest levels of education were no more likely to feel comfortable talking about this subject than was any other section of society. I found just as much interest, sympathy and understanding from such people as cleaners, policemen and bus drivers as from professors of psychology. Indeed, the former seemed less likely to talk in euphemisms. One intellectual group in London, having an interest in science and spirituality, kept laughing as I told my (as I thought sombre) story and this was most disconcerting. Maybe they were not sure how to react and this was some form of escape reaction.

I received a large number of letters, mainly from sufferers. For the most part they came from the UK but included France, Sweden, Eire, Canada and Australia. Men and women were about equally represented, as were all social classes. Some wrote by hand lengthy page after seemingly interminable page, including even the tiniest details of their lives. I was very touched by their pain and the concern of these people for me. Some wrote that they were praying for me. One man from Scotland accused me of Satanic and perverse sexuality. The single most common, indeed nearly universal, theme to emerge from these letters was something along the following lines:

'Thank you so much, since I know now that I am not alone. I feel part of a community and therefore not so odd. Reading about you made me feel better. The fact that you have this disorder and are successful makes me feel less peculiar.'

Some portrayed themselves as tortured souls who were misunderstood by friends and family alike. They felt totally alienated from the world and were desperate for some kind of empathy and validation as a person. A number just begged with me – please, please, tell me what to do, I can't stand this torment any longer! Each one among a significant number of letter-writers seemed genuinely to have believed that they were the only person in the world with the condition. At last, putting a name to it helped them. They could now go to their doctor and speak with greater confidence. Some reported that they had thrust the book under their doctors' noses and requested a prescription for a serotonin-reuptake inhibitor (described in Part 2). They added that they really had not felt confident in describing the condition before. Some said that they had been frightened to tell anyone about their condition and managed successfully to keep it from everyone's eyes.

Empathy with me was the greatest single feeling universally expressed. A man from Bognor Regis wrote:

'I could not understand how someone I had never met could write a book about me.'

And Francis from Fulham stated:

'It so clearly paralleled my own experience as to be quite uncanny!'

One woman wrote:

'There is something particularly fascinating about being granted an insight into someone else's inner mental life.'

A man revealed:

'I felt like an alien. It was very difficult to believe that there were other people out there who were experiencing the same problems as I was and the great depressing, rarely receding pain. Now I feel like part of a club. Albeit a very odd club.'

A man from Canada wrote, concerning his wife:

'Looking back, I find it very hard to understand how she could have put up with me all that time.'

A woman from Warwick told me:

'I never give up hope of freeing myself.'

The occasional person was shocked at how little professional help and understanding they had found, having been shunted around from one therapist to another. Some people reported that personal knowledge and contacts seemed to count for much. My feeling is that regional variations are great, London and Oxford probably being 'the best places' in England to have the disorder. A number expressed the hope that a greater public awareness of the condition would benefit all. Thus, a woman from Scotland wrote:

'I feel as if I am constantly battling against the professionals, just to get them to understand this illness and the severity of it. It seems to me that if you aint got a physical problem people can see and understand then you aint got a genuine problem.'

Similarly, from Teignmouth, a man informed me:

'In any other field of medicine one gets "referred to a specialist" if the condition is beyond local experience, but in this field there seems only to be a blank wall . . . yet one is aware that there is a whole industry of specialist people "out there" producing all the learned articles in the journals etc. but they seem to be surrounded by some moat to prevent "patients" from getting anywhere near them.'

Peter from Reading wrote:

'Whilst I am usually fairly articulate, I find that your book clearly exposes what I should have told my doctor over the years. I am now hoping that I can persuade him to read it as an aid to me helping myself.'

A large group of people asked me to give them contact details of specialists in their area, but alas I have never had this knowledge.
Ian from the Channel Islands wrote:

'This disorder must have an incredibly detrimental effect on intellectual performance, and it frightens me when I experience moments of low obsessional frequency as I realise my brain is much better than I usually give myself credit for. All that wasted ability!'

Actually this disorder and the personality type so commonly associated with it are by no means all bad news when it comes to creativity, as is discussed in Part 2.

There was an unusual case (unusual, that is, among the letters sent to me) of a woman from Dublin who complained about the anti-social behaviour of her obsessional partner, which could be classed as a case of abuse triggered by obsessional disorder:

> 'As he has always taken his frustrations out on me and managed to cover up for everybody else in social circles, everyone thought we were the ideal couple!! I am sure we could be quite a happy family if it was not for his problem.'

Some spoke of the difficulty they experienced in going public, Pat, from Sherbourne, being among these:

> 'I've found that telling people about my condition makes them not want to know me, so I now shut up about it.'

Some expressed great relief to know that they were not psychotic – not 'mad' in the traditional sense of the word. A woman wrote to me from Hampshire, speaking on behalf of her self-help group:

> 'Our group now refers to you as 'Fred', as I hope you don't mind us calling you, and wish to congratulate you on your most interesting and comforting dialogue. We, as a group, know that we are not alone and are definitely not "mad".'

A woman from Carlisle wrote an inspirational message:

> 'What struck me when reading your book was how we can make something positive come out of even the most horrible experiences.'

Some of the people writing to me were keen to establish a personal rapport in the form of pointing out shared star-signs, having learned to speak the same foreign languages or also having been born in the vicinity of Cambridge. One woman sent me a copy of my book with all of the sections highlighted that applied most to her.

Looking through the letters, it was clear that for a very significant number the disorder was either triggered or strongly exacerbated by stresses in their lives, such as unemployment, alcoholism, suicide of a relative or marital difficulties. One woman reported that it was when her husband was on heroin that her obsessions were at their worst. Several people wrote that they were motivated to 'get to the bottom of it all' and I responded that this might not prove to be an effective approach.

On a rather lighter note, some people would make a remark such as 'I know what you mean. My husband is strongly obsessional. He needs to spend every weekend either watching football or fishing.' I would then suggest that this was a quite different phenomenon from what I was talking about and would ask them, 'Does he resist this? Would he find it appropriate to seek medical help, say, in the form of tablets?' That was usually enough to convince them that their husband was not an obsessional in the sense used here.

A large number of apparently healthy people would come up to me to tell me in private about their particular and serious obsessions. Open University (OU) students at summer school were a major source of such information. Others reported brief periods of, say, obsessional checking but these episodes went away without causing too much distress: 'We know what it must be like'. This highlights the fact that there are not always neat boundaries between normality and illness.

Kathy, an OU psychology student and friend from Hertfordshire, wrote to me:

> 'Lots of people who don't actually suffer nevertheless feel that they have odd little impulses which they feel compelled to follow from time to time – like not standing on cracks in the pavement. I always like my old teddy bear to be facing me when I get into bed at night; if it's slipped or is facing the wall I feel that it will "mind". Ridiculous!'

Somewhat alarmingly, two people (one being a policeman and OU student, the other an OU secretary) told me that their obsessions had been triggered by reading about them in my book. They added that, mercifully, these experiences did not last too long.

I was invited to address self-help groups and was overwhelmed by the participants' desperation to get better, desire to understand the nature of their disorder and their empathy towards me. I found these experiences moving but profoundly depressing and draining. There seemed to be some limit to the amount of all this that I felt I could take.

On occasions, it seemed that some sufferers were treating me as a kind of guru. One day the OU security staff were searching campus for me because a man had arrived at reception, burst into tears and refused to go until I met him. The staff at reception were frightened at what might happen next. By the time someone found me and walked with me to reception, he was sitting on the grass and still crying. He turned out to be an engine-driver (a vocation always very near to my own heart!), who had driven down to Milton Keynes from Manchester. I had a long talk with him about both obsessions and our shared love of trains and then he left, still very distressed. I felt worried about him, and often wonder where he is now and hope that he is feeling better (driving his engine through Milton Keynes at 100 mph?).

Even in the context of obsessionality, humour can also enter the picture. For example, it might surprise some people to know that the self-help group meetings were not always entirely sombre tearful occasions for 100 per cent of the time. Occasionally someone would register some irony and humour in their behaviour and cathartic applause would break out.

At one meeting in south London, a man approached me – 'I have been married for 30 years but I keep having these thoughts that I could kill my wife. Tell me, please – am I really evil or just obsessional?' The audience seemed to really like this question. I was well aware of the dangers of reassurance to a patient who might be undergoing exposure therapy, so I said: 'I will tell you just once and *only once* that you are obsessional and not evil". I just had to hope that this might give a kick-start to some kind of mental reorganisation.

The next day in the OU restaurant, I met an old friend, Richard, a well-known and much-loved university character and comic, alas no longer with us on this Earth. He asked me how I got on at the meeting and I told him about the question concerning evil or obsessionality. Richard disagreed entirely with my analysis: 'I would have told him that he is neither evil nor obsessional – on the contrary, to my way of thinking anyone who has been married for 30 years and *doesn't* have the regular thought that they could kill their partner has probably got something rather wrong with them!' Richard was speaking 'slightly' in jest but the example might be used to illustrate the serious and important point that the definition of obsessionality cannot be made in terms of the thought content on its own. Rather, it is the individual's interpretation and pain level associated with the thought that is an essential ingredient of any diagnosis.

After speaking at a meeting of the OU Students' Association in Manchester, a woman came up to me and said that I had saved her life. She had made the firm decision to commit suicide but my book gave her the hope that she might be cured, which she now was. When this kind of comment appeared again, it 'went to my head' and I was engaged with feelings of my own self-importance. I was brought back to reality by the thought that personnel, say, of the fire, nursing or ambulance services might be told exactly the same thing – not just two or three times but every day!

Sometimes I would arrange to meet the more serious cases. I would end the phone call saying something like 'So, see you under the departure board at Euston at 3 p.m. on this Friday.' Perhaps somewhat predictably, they would then ring back to ask 'Was it really this Friday?' or 'Is there only one departure board at Euston?'

I was most impressed by the ingenuity of some sufferers and their families. A woman from Didcot suggested exploiting modern technology and using a 'virtual world' method to help sufferers to gain exposure to their feared object (they might wear goggles onto which programmed images could be presented). For example, someone might gain virtual exposure to contamination and be allowed to wash their hands virtually but for only a limited and programmed time. This time would decrease over days of exposure.

Another clever idea emerged when I was on a phone-in at Radio Leicester. A man told me of the plan that he and his wife had just devised to help him complete his checks. They had produced a board with a series of numbered spaces on it. These corresponded to the numbers of the targets of each evening's check – for example, 1 would be the gas taps and 2 would be the toilet window. Then just before retiring, the wife would attach a series of numbered sticky labels to the targets. The man would then do his rounds, peel the labels off in sequence and attach them to the corresponding space on the board, after he had ascertained that all was well at each target. The end of checking would be indicated by covering of the spaces on the board, which could then be taken like a trophy to the bedroom and presented to the wife.

He asked what I thought – would it be likely to work? I pointed out the infinite diversity of human variation and experience. What gives the necessary feedback and peace of mind to one individual might trigger new complex layers of obsessionality in another. There would probably be no harm done in trying it and the wife could prove invaluable in guiding this activity. However, if the technique failed and he then found he needed a second board and back-up series of labels, his wife was in great danger of being drawn into just a new variant of the ritual. She should carefully monitor her husband's behaviour and strongly resist any such temptation.

I felt a strong sense of responsibility on these phone-ins but a very limited power to help. For example, on a national radio interview, a woman said that she had been travelling regularly each week from Norwich to London for psychoanalysis. Would I recommend her continuation of this course of action? I told her that quite honestly I could not recommend it. However, I realised that most probably she was then lost to me in terms of any follow-up advice.

A number of therapists contacted me, some with radically different interpretations from my own. This made for a fruitful exchange of ideas. Barbara, a therapist from Brighton, wrote:

'Hearing one client, just yesterday, tell his intrusive, unwanted thought, "you can be there if you like but you have no power over me" is perhaps one of the most deeply satisfying experiences I have ever shared with anybody.'

A couple of scientific papers from Cambridge and London reported testing of the technique described by me to gain unique feedback on each day's check (described in Part 2).

The book also gave me my first experience of performing 'informal therapy', after I acquired an obsessional flat-mate. I met Mary (not her real name), who was 25 years old and from York, when I was giving a talk in Birmingham. Mary was hospitalised at that time to protect her from very serious compulsive hand-washing rituals. The skin had been peeled from her hands by the washing. She later rang me up and asked if she might come and stay with me. I talked to the nurse in charge of the ward and she explained to me that Mary was getting nowhere being hospitalised. Rather, Mary needed to be reintegrated into the community (cynics told me to read this as 'we would love to get rid of her').

Mary had a figure like a fashion model and, despite obsessions about sexuality, took no steps to disguise it. I am sure that some people must have thought that I had an ulterior motive in 'acquiring' her but I didn't. My girl-friend at the time used Mary as a reason to terminate the relationship, though other reasons were also involved. She told me I was truly mad to take such a gamble – 'suppose that she accuses you of rape?' In reality, Mary never accused me of anything, just as I felt she would not.

Mary explained that she was obsessed by sexual contamination, which could be gained from towels or even from an infected person passing the flat at a distance. She showed a clear class bias in her fears. A scruffy appearance was definitely correlated with an increased fear of contamination. Sexually expressive dressing by women was a particular target for triggering her obsessions, in spite of the fact that Mary's appearance in itself caused male drivers to turn their heads and stare. When we were out together, Mary was constantly scanning the path for any sign of a condom left behind and could richly imagine almost any object to be one.

In Mary's way of seeing things, only by means of extensive washing rituals could she be protected from contamination. After the washing, Mary needed to cover herself in oil, wrap a towel around her body and run to the bedroom. On one occasion, a good friend Quentin came to the door just as Mary was doing her run and thereby the dreaded contamination was let in. That evening's extensive ritual was immediately declared null and void and had to be started all over again, much to Quentin's amazement.

Mary washed for enormous periods of time and would only use a towel once. She needed then to wash this towel, which she would only do by hand, thereby getting into a vicious circle. I did not have a washing machine then and used the communal one in our block of flats. Mary would not use this for fear of contamination. Not surprisingly, she soon ran out of towels and asked to borrow one of mine. I didn't say anything but wondered how the obvious conflict among fears could possibly be resolved. The answer was soon to come. Mary asked how long the towel had been in my flat since it had been washed and I said about two weeks. She suggested that this was long enough for it to be decontaminated by the atmosphere of the flat. As long as Mary was in a hermetically sealed and trusted environment, she seemed to be protected from the dreaded and contaminated world out there. Alas, it didn't do much to help the state of damp of the flat!

At first, Mary sank into very low spirits and told me she wanted to kill herself: 'I just do not understand how anyone could have a dread or a fear of death. This is ridiculous. Death must be great since it gets you out of all this crap. Just give me the courage to do it.' (One obsessional often has inordinate difficulty understanding what is alarming about the content of another obsessional's thought, though they can invariably empathise with the form that the thoughts take.) One day, I returned home from university to find Mary in the kitchen holding a bread-knife. She was patting the blade on the arteries of her arm while looking at me, saying nothing. I was terrified but felt that a rational argument might only be counter-productive, so I decided to take the coward's way out: 'Mary, please don't do it here. If you must, please go somewhere else.' She then put the knife away.

I decided that I would try some behavioural psychology. Mary had just expressed a love for the somewhat sugary music of the group named The Carpenters and an admiration for Karen Carpenter. 'Oh, my God – please don't let her become anorexic like Karen Carpenter, too!', I thought but decided it was worth a try. I was going shopping later in the day and suggested that I buy a video of this duo. Being safely out of earshot of highbrow OU intellectuals, I was prepared to admit to Mary that I too liked the sound of The Carpenters. I made a deal with her: for every 10 minutes less she spent bathing at night, so we would watch 10 minutes of The Carpenters. This worked up to a point, a testimony to the power of behavioural psychology.

I learned just how difficult it can be to live with an obsessional. I had the strength of theoretical conviction towards a behavioural psychological approach and felt that I gave good advice to others. However, at times I caught myself falling back on the kind of naïve home-spun wisdom that is useless at best, if not dangerously counter-productive. Without giving any thought to it, I would say something like 'Mary, you really must try harder for my sake.' I would then recall my swimming teacher at school giving me similar advice – 'If you want to swim, don't do that. You will never swim unless you try harder.' Absolutely useless is such advice – I still cannot swim – but alas it has a certain compelling and intuitive attraction.

With the help of a good friend, Madeline, and a local headmaster, we managed to get Mary active in the local community by helping in a school. Mary was very good at this and showed a real talent for getting on with children. On one occasion, we were asked for lunch at Madeline's home and arrived by bus, after some shopping in the city centre. Madeline had not quite got the salad ready and asked us to help with this and to cut some bread, etc. We both noticed with some shock that, without bothering to wash her hands first, Mary launched straight into touching food. It is amazing as just how selectively focused the contents of obsessional thoughts can be and how they can run counter to any conventional logic.

The last that I heard of Mary was that she had moved to Wales and was living with a psychiatric nurse, Bill. Bill had been caring for Mary and this was how the relationship developed.

Apart from acquiring Mary and losing my girlfriend, the period from the appearance of the book in 1990 to 1993 passed without any dramatic changes in my life. Then in 1993 in Bucharest, I met Olga, a Romanian, to whom I got married and who is the co-author of this

2nd edition of the book. It was love at first sight and from then we have never looked back. I acquired a son, Stanislav, a gifted musician, and an ex-Soviet Doberman, named Pinta Ben Thelma.

Olga was from Moldova (formerly a republic of the Soviet Union), a fascinating part of the world and, at the time of writing, the poorest country in Europe. If ever both the strength of love for a woman and a loyalty to railways were put to the test, it was surely in making journeys between Bucharest and the Moldovan capital, Chisinau, a 15-hour trek. Four hours are spent at the frontier of the old USSR, where an endless stream of uniformed men come to shine torches and inspect both you and the compartment. Then they need to change all of the wheels on the train to accommodate the different gauge. This part of the world is definitely not for the faint-hearted. I will spare you the details of life on an ex-Soviet train, as one sees enough in one journey to trigger a lifetime of obsessional thoughts. Now there are international flight links with the West and a superb new airport terminal building.

Romania was a very hospitable country in which to spend a period as a guest professor, and the time in Moldova with Olga's family was wonderful. This is a part of the world very gifted linguistically. People might not have much in the way of material possessions but they certainly know how to make the most of what they have. Even the poorest of families knows how to put on a sumptuous banquet for guests and the wine flows very freely – alas, too freely for me on several occasions. Cut off from e-mail, fax and telephone, and with an orchard nearby, it was an ideal location in which to do serious academic work.

The former Communist world of Eastern Europe is surely one of the most odd places on Earth. Because of the severe winter, the university in Bucharest had no working public toilet. As a special guest, I was allowed to collect a key for the one working 'VIP toilet', inaccessible to students. I never did find out what they did if nature were suddenly to call. My lectures were in English except for one spot of ten minutes in French. The reason for this shift of languages was simple: the interpreter had got stuck in the snow. I asked the students whether anyone else could interpret from English and in so far as they understood the question they said 'no'. Then a woman whom I had not seen before asked if I knew French. If I did, she was prepared to interpret from French to Romanian for me. Then after ten minutes of French, the snow-clad interpreter arrived. Afterwards I thanked the woman and asked why I had not seen her before. She replied 'I am no part of this course but a student of the Czech language. I am only here to take notes for my boyfriend who is ill.' This did not stop her participating fully and intelligently in the discussion, which perhaps says something about psychology as a subject.

In 1997, I achieved another great excitement of my life. I had been invited by an old friend Kent Berridge to the University of Michigan at Ann Arbor (just outside Detroit) to give a special guest lecture supported by a series of student tutorials. Ann Arbor is a most beautiful town and Kent took us to visit the Tamla Motown museum in Detroit, the house where the original hits of the Supremes and the Temptations, among many others, were recorded (this obsessional has an insatiable appetite for nostalgia). Alas, in Detroit, I thought I must be getting old or this is the most polite place on earth, or both. For the first time in my life, in a bar two men got up and offered me their seats!

By coincidence, just before leaving England, I had at last established contact details of the agent's office for the original Lettermen, my pop-idols from the early years. The passing decades had done nothing to dent my enthusiasm for this sound. One day, when ringing their office, I found myself on the phone to Jim Pike, a founder member of the group, quite unaware that it was he. Only when I asked for his name did I find out who he was. When I discovered this, I was not quite sure what to say but I can only guess that it was not too foolish since he invited Olga and me to meet the group. We established that their nearest concert to Detroit at that time was in San Francisco, not exactly just around the corner! Nevertheless, we flew there, went to the concert and afterwards were taken out by the group for a meal in a Greek restaurant. This was an unforgettable experience. I was struck by just how 'simple' (in the best sense of the word) and down to earth these guys were; they seemed keener to talk about such things as psychology in the Open University than their own music.

By an amazing coincidence, during the meal I also discovered that group member Bob Engemann was the nephew of Norbert Weiner. Weiner is the father of the science of cybernetics (the study of how insights from systems theory and engineering can illuminate psychology and the brain). As a 23-year-old Lettermen fan, I had read his classic *Cybernetics* in the YMCA hostel in New York City and my life's research had been strongly influenced by such thinking. Bob asked me to explain briefly what on Earth Uncle Norbert had been going on about and this I managed to do. I suspect that any pedagogical skills I exhibited were more impressive to them than my musical talents. Thus, when they asked me what is my favourite Lettermen hit song I must have got the title wrong, as they didn't recognise it. Worse still, I tried to sing it to them and they still couldn't recognise it!

Looking back over events in their lives, obsessionals are probably no less prone to cringes of embarrassment than are the rest of the population (probably more so) and I certainly am very prone. Dear reader, just try to imagine what it is like to recall singing in vain in a San Francisco restaurant to a team voted by *Billboard* as the world's best vocal harmony group. Enough of that, I can't stand it!

The obsessions were at a low level and the technique of 'brain lock', pioneered by Jeffrey Schwartz of Los Angeles, was proving useful. In this, one simply tries to reattribute any obsessions to a malfunction in the brain, a technique described in detail in the next part of the book.

If you are a sufferer from obsessional disorder you should certainly not be discouraged after reading this first section of the book. Although no treatment provides a 100% guarantee, there is still room for you to feel that appropriate help is available and there is a good chance that something will work for you. It is true that for me no single treatment seemed to provide a solution to the problem. However, I did in the end improve. Also, I strongly suspect that I was a particularly difficult case to treat.

Part 2
What is obsessional disorder and what can be done about it?

11
The nature of the problem

Obsessive compulsive disorder (or obsessional compulsive disorder) – abbreviated as OCD – presents a peculiar challenge and often formidable difficulty not only for the individual affected but also for the doctor, psychiatrist and researcher, as well as friends and family. It consists of unwanted and intrusive thoughts often (but not always) accompanied by behaviour that has an element of compulsion to it. It is often very hard indeed for the 'normal' person to appreciate just how much distress is caused by obsessional disorder. For such activities as *checking*, people are tempted to apply simple rationality – why don't you stop? Worse still, the behaviour can evoke the response – 'Snap out of it' or 'Pull yourself together'. But, in the extreme, the problem can be every bit as difficult to cope with and as debilitating as any other mental disorder.

Some notable investigators have studied obsessional disorder; for example, Sigmund Freud (1856–1939), and the distinguished French psychologist Pierre Janet (1859–1947), who made a meticulous and extensive study of obsessionals in Paris. Janet is relatively unknown in the English-speaking world. His classic work on the subject of obsessionality, *Les Obsessions et la Psychasthénie*, has never been translated into English. This has been a great loss to psychology. Because French is no longer a natural second language in the English-speaking world, researchers and therapists often have, at best, only second-hand knowledge of Janet's work. His book is beautifully written in a simple unaffected style, with a maximum of sympathy for his patients and their own insight, and with a minimum of unsupported speculation. His theoretical speculations were always modestly made, with extensive reference to the work of earlier researchers.

Freud, a rather different personality type from Janet, had a strong interest in OCD, and two of his most famous cases, those of 'Wolf-man' and 'The Rat Man', were apparently obsessionals. There is some suggestion that Freud himself had experience of the obsessional phenomenon, and he certainly believed that it would be a very fruitful area to investigate in the future. Unfortunately, psychoanalytical techniques have not lived up to this promise, although some features of the disorder are often well described in the psychoanalytic literature.

Exactly what is obsessional disorder?

What are obsessional experiences and who has them? It is difficult to describe exactly what an obsessional disorder is but perhaps not so hard as for the diagnosis of other mental disorders. There is fairly good agreement as to its definition and diagnosis, possibly better than for, say, schizophrenia.

Obsessional thoughts consist of a mental image or idea that has a feeling of *compulsion* or *imposition* – often associated with an inner pressure to make affected people perform actions that run counter to a rational intention. The obsessive quality of the thought overrides any resistance that the individual can offer. The thoughts are perceived as alien and often perverse, bizarre or morbid. (It is often possible to detect a change of heart rate when the unwanted thought is experienced.) The person tends to be brooding and doubting, and given to speculation about the significance of the thoughts. For example, the individual might speculate that they are a sign that harm will come unless some particular action (e.g. washing or checking) is taken.

A major problem with obsessions that are not accompanied by bizarre behaviour is that, by definition, the disorder cannot be observed by others. Indeed, the person's behaviour might look amazingly normal. On the other hand, where compulsive behaviour is concerned, this is often either checking or *washing*. A person might wash his hands for hours on end in an attempt to purify them or to prevent harm to others. Such behaviour is easy to define and measure. Although bizarre, the behaviour is not morally unacceptable, and so, with some coaxing and reassurance, one might expect to be able to extract fairly truthful accounts from the individual.

Because they are usually meticulous and articulate, obsessional people can often provide their doctor with reliable information about their behaviour. My own (F.T.'s) doctor once told me that he would like to be able to test all of his new drugs on me! It is interesting, though, that Pierre Janet reported great trouble in getting his patients to confess the truth about their thoughts. These days, as in Janet's time, patients are sometimes simply too embarrassed to 'come clean' and speak the truth. They prefer to skate around the central problem, discussing only such things as 'general unease' or 'low spirits'. However, it is extremely important to be as honest as possible, as soon as possible. Knowing that others suffer from, say, unacceptable sexual or violent thoughts can be a source of comfort and will speed the 'opening up'. Once under care, obsessionals are generally good patients and, having started on a course of treatment, tend to see it through conscientiously. On the other hand, the doctor runs the risk of being inundated with both spoken and written information from the patient.

What *is* and *is not* an obsessional disorder

The common use of the word 'obsession' is distinct from both an *obsessional personality* (one prone to extremes of trying to gain control, perfectionism and persistence) and an *obsessive compulsive disorder* (OCD). We commonly describe people as 'obsessional' without their so-called obsession being a problem to them. For instance, great inventors and scientists are often described as 'obsessed' with their intellectual challenge. They might *ruminate* (mentally 'chew over') about a particular idea in a repetitive manner for years on end, before finding a solution. The great composers, such as Schumann, vividly described the endless toil that is necessary to achieve perfection. Our lives are richer as a result of such dogged persistence. These are mental and behavioural phenomena rather different from what are meant by the expressions 'obsessional thoughts' and 'obsessional behaviour'. In OCD we are concerned with phenomena that seriously trouble the subject. By stark contrast, Schumann didn't resist his musical thoughts; on the contrary, they were part of his calling.

Some people might be described as being obsessed with seeking sex or the pursuit of money. However, this is not an obsessional problem or disorder. These individuals are not driven that way to neutralise an unpleasant intrusive thought. The more usual erotic thoughts might well be distracting or frustrating but would not normally be considered unpleasantly intrusive. In the present context, enjoyable thoughts or impulses are not 'obsessional'.

Neither is the spontaneous and unprovoked nature of a thought sufficient to classify it as a problem. Both Beethoven and Mozart described how some of their creative ideas just came from 'nowhere'. Going from the sublime to the ridiculous, I (F.T.) am sure that I am no exception in frequently having just one line of a current pop song on my mind for ages and being 'compelled' to sing it. This certainly causes no pain to me; indeed, I greatly enjoy it, though I can't speak for those within earshot!

Consider the man who used to spend each day standing at Oxford Circus in London with a banner proclaiming 'Eat less protein. Protein stimulates sexual passion.' He might have been said by some to be obsessed with his eccentric cause. In this context, the term has pejorative connotations, implying that his time might have been better spent doing something more fruitful. However, he was not behaving as an obsessional neurotic, because he did not resist his calling. The behaviour fitted his life's goals. It would be inappropriate in a free society to suggest that he might have considered changing his behaviour or have needed psychiatric help.

The everyday use of the word 'obsession' has a vivid meaning, and presumably people will go on employing it in this sense. We simply need to take care not to include, for example, the dedicated scientist or police officer or the religious fanatic when considering the subject at a medical level. To contrast the common usage of 'obsession' with our true quarry, obsessional disorder, consider the intrusive thoughts described by John Bunyan, which acted against his life's purpose:

> '. . . if I have been hearing the Word, then uncleanliness, blasphemies, and despair, would hold me as Captive there; if I have been reading, then sometimes I had sudden thoughts to question all I read; sometimes again my mind would be so strangely snatched away, and possessed with other things, that I have neither known, nor regarded, nor remembered so much as the sentence that but now I have read.
>
> 'Sometimes again, when I have been preaching, I have been violently assaulted with thoughts of blasphemy, and strongly tempted to speak them with my mouth before the Congregation.'

These thoughts vividly illustrate the technically or medically correct use of the term 'obsessional disorder'.

The dictionary definition of obsession is somewhat nearer the medical usage. The origin of the word is the Latin *obsidere*, which means 'to besiege'. Definitions of the verb 'to obsess' generally involve 'to beset', 'to assail', 'to possess', 'to harass like a besieging force or an evil spirit'. The *Oxford English Dictionary* shows a significant change of emphasis between the early and late 17th century. Compare the following two definitions of 'obsession':

'The hostile action of the devil or an evil spirit besetting any one; actuation by the devil or an evil spirit from without; the fact of being thus beset or actuated',

and

'The action of any influence, notion or "fixed idea" which persistently assails or vexes, especially so as to discompose the mind'.

Coming to more recent times, *Chambers Concise Dictionary* captures an aspect of obsessional rumination in its definition of obsession as 'morbid persistence of an idea in the mind, against one's will; a fixed idea'.

Our usage of 'obsession' conforms to the definition given by Graham Reed, as applied to someone who constantly has '. . . intrusive and persistent mental events [thoughts], which he usually recognises as being foolish and unacceptable but which, despite all his efforts, he is unable to dispel'.

The meaning of obsession that we use here emphasises the unwelcome nature of the intrusion, that these thoughts are in some sense imposed upon the conscious mind against its wishes. An accurate definition will help us to distinguish the condition from other distinct disorders that have some characteristics in common with it. Repetitive mental events, even associated with repetitive movements, are found in a variety of disorders that would not be called obsessional, such as schizophrenia and some diseases of the nervous system. This is a vital consideration for a doctor providing a diagnosis. If the person realises that the thoughts causing the trouble are senseless or illogical, this can be a valuable indication of the existence of an obsessional problem, but such realisation should not be regarded as a necessary condition. In 1938, Sir Aubrey Lewis said:

'Critical appraisal of the obsession and recognition that it is absurd represents a defensive, intellectual effort, intended to destroy it: it is not always present, nor is the obsessional idea always absurd.'

For Lewis the crucial ingredient was that the individual tries to resist or destroy the thought. We prefer to say that the individual initially opposes the thought but, after a very long while, might simply give up the struggle.

We are concerned therefore with thoughts that are frequent, unpleasant and, in general, resisted. Certain wanted and pleasant thoughts might sometimes appear to invade our consciousness.

However, these are not classed here as 'obsessional' because they are wanted and are not resisted. For practical purposes, we can rule out the experience of occasional unpleasant intrusive thoughts as being obsessional. A survey carried out on London students showed that most of them experienced thoughts, both positive and negative, that were perceived as intruding. The thought content often did not differ very much from that of people with obsessional disorder. What distinguished these so-called 'normal' thoughts from those creating a serious problem was that the abnormal obsessional thoughts:

- last longer,

- are more intense and occur more frequently,

- are perceived as more alien and accompanied by stronger urges to neutralisation (the attempt to find a thought that counters the intrusion),

- are resisted more strongly,

- are harder to dismiss.

Similarly, many people have small rituals that they feel the need to observe. These are, of course, quite different from OCD that disrupts one's life.

It is interesting that obsessional people can evoke their unwanted thought on demand more easily than can 'normal' people. The thought has a low threshold – it is easily triggered – as though it is permanently on 'stand-by', ready to come to the surface. In this very limited respect, obsessional people could, paradoxically, be said to have more control of their thought content than do others.

To summarise, obsessional thoughts are regarded as deserving treatment because of their quality, frequency and the resistance that they evoke.

How many people have the disorder?

In the past, some estimates reckoned that as many as 1–2 per cent of the US population had some form or other of an obsessional problem. The latest estimate is that in the UK and the USA some 2–3 per cent of the population will have the disorder at some time during their life. Some 50 million people in the world today appear to suffer from it. An even larger percentage suffers from so-called 'subclinical obsession' –

a mild version not justifying intervention. The chances are that everyone knows well at least one person with the condition. However, the number of patients complaining primarily of obsessional disorders is not a large percentage of those receiving psychiatric care (something like 3 per cent of people treated for neuroses), so it is possible that someone seeking medical help could find themselves to be their doctor's first patient with this condition. And so the doctor might be unsure about appropriate therapy or medication. Giving a precise figure for the incidence of the disorder, based on the number of people seeking psychiatric help, is almost impossible because of the overlap of obsessional disorder with other conditions, such as anorexia nervosa, panic disorder, phobias and depression.

Obsessionals are more secretive than other people with psychological problems and so it is the more serious disorders that tend to get seen by the medical profession. Without doubt, very many simply suffer in silence. Sometimes even people with severe problems seek medical attention only after heavy persuasion from relatives or close friends. It is common for them to endure the condition for years before they seek help.

Nature and nurture

What do these terms mean?

The term 'nature' describes what we acquire at the point of our conception, whereas 'nurture' refers to the environment to which we are exposed. Sometimes questions are posed as to which of them is the more important but such questions are fundamentally misleading. Without genes there is no life and without an environment there is no life. Both are needed to develop a human, and weight cannot be given to one against the other. However, we can ask intelligently whether differences between people are due to differences in genes or environment.

So, is OCD inherited? It is commonly argued in the scientific literature that it is. The illness is relatively common among the relatives of obsessionals. Given the argument on nature and nurture that has just been made, what exactly is meant by such a condition 'being inherited'? The term refers to the genes that people inherit from their parents. Some disorders are known to be inherited in the sense that the offspring are bound to acquire the condition if one or both of the parents have it. OCD is not like this in that there is no such certainty about its inheritance. Obsessional disorder can occur in children whose parents and grandparents had no sign of it. Conversely, obsessional parents might have children with no subsequent sign of the disorder. The scientific evidence suggests only that a *tendency* to the condition is transmitted genetically between generations.

An analogy could prove useful here. Suppose that a piece of glass is said to be brittle. This means that it has a strong *tendency* to break, given a certain stress. It does not mean that it will necessarily break. Conversely, describing another piece of glass as non-brittle does not mean that it will never break. This analogy makes an important general point about nature and nurture, or genes and environment: the outcome of their action is a complex interdependence. Things are not 'either/or' or 'one or the other' but an interaction of the two. Knowing that there is a genetic contribution to the disorder in no sense plays down the importance of the environment.

So, perhaps the most common reason for the appearance of OCD is in terms of such a genetically inherited tendency ('predisposition') to the disorder combined with a trigger event ('precipitating event'). Some people with OCD worry that any children they have will inherit the disorder. They might take comfort from the lack of a very close association between genes and the disorder and from the current success of treatments. Researchers are learning more all the time. Also, such parents can always try to do all in their power to reduce the chances of the child being affected.

Researching the question

What is the evidence that scientists use to claim that this disorder is inherited? One standard research tool is to compare identical and non-identical ('fraternal') twins. Identical twins derive from a single fertilised egg and are therefore genetically identical. Fraternal twins derive from two fertilised eggs and, although genetically similar, are not identical. So, suppose that Bill and Ben are identical twins and Bill has the disorder. If there is a strong genetic contribution, we might suppose that the chances are that Ben will also have it. If Jack and Dick are also identical twins and Jack has no signs of the disorder, we might expect Dick not to have it either. In other words, we would expect the *concordance* of the disorder to be relatively high between identical twins. It should be less strong among fraternal twins and indeed this is precisely what is found.

Of course, identical twins might be treated more similarly than fraternal twins and this could explain their higher concordance. For this reason researchers seek twins who have been adopted into different families. Still the leads point to a genetic contribution to OCD.

Upbringing and imitation

Might the tendencies be passed on by children imitating their parents? Again it is difficult to make the necessary observations, but imitation of specific behaviours seems unlikely to happen often. Imitating strategies for dealing with the world – such as timidity and caution – seems to be more likely. By genetics or by environmental observation, or more likely a subtle interaction of the two, the child might well come to acquire a tendency to timidity and over-dependence. Some experts would regard this as fertile soil for the later development of obsessional disorder. The home environment of obsessionals tends to be excessively controlled. However, the number of obsessionals coming from 'perfectly normal' backgrounds makes any simple and unqualified appeal to 'faulty upbringing' suspicious. Parents should not blame themselves!

Age of onset

Obsessional disorder usually reveals itself between the ages of 20 and 30 years, though obsessional patients often report a variety of neurotic symptoms (or 'over-sensitivity') in childhood. Adult obsessional patients often experience phobias (exaggerated fears of particular things such as heights or spiders) and mild compulsions in childhood. Obsessional traits are also common before the full-blown disorder emerges, although this is by no means always so.

Full-blown obsessional disorder is also found in children. As noted above, this can happen even where there is neither indication of obsessional personality before the disorder develops nor evidence of obsessionality in the parents. Dr Jeffrey M Schwartz of Los Angeles has observed that children with OCD are sometimes able to tyrannise the family into conforming to the dictates of the child's compulsions. Parents often comply partly because they feel a sense of guilty responsibility for having brought the child into the world.

The average age at which professional help is sought is around 28 (F.T. was 29), though there might have been considerable trouble for years before this. It is rare to find the onset beyond the age of 40. Most of Janet's patients were between 20 and 40. Some investigators see the significance of the age factor as being that onset is rare outside what might be termed the active and striving period of life. The course of the trouble is sometimes up and down, commonly with two really bad periods in a lifetime. Stress or fatigue is likely to make the condition worse. For others the intensity of the problem is nearer constant, sometimes for life.

Is onset associated with a particular event?

According to a survey in Sweden, obsessionals can sometimes accurately date the time that their symptoms began (time of onset). For one patient, a pregnant woman, they began while she was cleaning fish. Holding the dead fish seemed to be the cue to provoke thoughts of the temporary nature of life. Another woman was mincing meat and became obsessed with the thought that she could mince the flesh of her husband. The onset was quite often associated with trauma that caused symptoms of great anxiety, such as abnormal breathing or activity of the heart. This anxiety could be caused by, for example, the death of someone close to the individual. However, for some people there might have been a bodily disturbance with no obvious cause, such as the feeling that they would stop breathing.

Also represented among patients trying to date the time of onset were temperature stress (being exposed to some extreme of temperature), a particular occasion involving excessive consumption of alcohol, pregnancy and abortion, and sexual and marital problems. Some investigators report that the precipitating factor occasionally involves unexpressed anger. In other cases, it is not easy to determine the precise age when the disorder began, because it was gradual. In 30–50 per cent of cases no precipitating event could be found. In some cases, obsessional disorders arise during the course of depression and outlast the depression itself.

The nature of the thoughts

The essence of the problem is that the thoughts are alien to the person's lifestyle, his or her ambitions and desires in life. They can disrupt work and pleasure alike. Affected people are unable to relax and accept the thought as irrelevant to their life. They usually feel compelled to resist it in some way. Their reactions and responses are likely to be much the same even after years of innumerable repetitions of the same theme.

For someone to be diagnosed as having an obsessive disorder it is crucial that the thoughts are unwanted by that person. Without this, even the content of the thoughts cannot be used unambiguously to identify an obsessional problem. For example, consider an individual whose problem consists of ruminating over why God created the world. Of course, some of the greatest intellects in history have occupied themselves with just that type of question but they would not necessarily be described as having psychiatric problems! What to them evoked pleasant awe, reverence, fascination and welcome challenge would, by contrast, torment the obsessional person.

Imagine two men experiencing the identical set of thoughts – that they are worthless individuals. The one man might indeed feel that he is one of life's failures and do nothing to resist the thoughts. The second might resist the thoughts, recognising that they are totally at odds with the true assessment of his worth. Only the second would be characterised as having an obsessional problem.

Although obsessional thoughts occur spontaneously, without prompting from outside, they can also be provoked by certain factors or events (e.g. passing a cemetery). Most obsessionals who seek treatment are easily able to trigger the obsessional thought in response to instructions from their therapist. This is important if treatment requires the person to consider the obsessional thought. By contrast, once raised, it is difficult to dismiss the thought, and the length of the time it persists seems to give some indication of the severity of the discomfort that the intrusions cause. A radical change of environment can sometimes produce temporary relief from obsessions. New signals from a different environment may inhibit the well-established obsessional signals in the brain.

The amount of resistance that obsessionals can muster in response to an intrusion will normally vary over time. Their 'will-power' fluctuates. The following are typical reports from obsessionals:

- 'I've been fighting it today, using all my will-power. Last week, I just didn't feel up to it.'

- 'I usually struggle with it. Today, I just feel too exhausted.'

- Another was able to escape from his ruminations after receiving news of promotion. 'I just feel on top of the world. I could handle anything . . .'

- One woman was particularly vulnerable during her menstrual period and when she had bowel trouble. 'There's too much stacked against me . . . It's bad enough fighting it at the best of times, but right now I feel helpless – I haven't the will-power to go on.'

Content of obsessional thoughts

Obsessional thoughts that do not involve compulsive behaviour can, to a large extent, be divided into three categories: religious, sexual and violent.

Religious obsessional thoughts

These seem to be somewhat less common now than was the case in the past, as might be expected from the decline in influence of the Christian church in the UK. At one time the condition now called 'obsessional disorder' was described as religious melancholy, indicating its likeness to what we now call 'depression'. A typical obsession of this class (if any obsession can be described as 'typical') might be the fear of shouting 'Jesus is a bastard' in church on Sunday. Affected people might feel a 'behavioural impulse': for example, that they are about to shout obscenities in a public place, and feel themselves resisting this impulse.

Pierre Janet encountered a relatively large number of patients with this kind of obsession. Their thoughts were a mix of sacred and profane aspects: examples included thoughts of a soul contaminated by excrement and a sexual perversion committed in church. For years, Claire, one of Janet's patients, had experienced about 200 times a day the intrusive thought of a penis and the bread of holy communion. In some cases, months passed before a patient would tell Janet the true nature of their thoughts. In the meantime, doctor and patient would go round in circles getting no nearer than discussing vague versions of the central theme. Such patients often had a history of spending time in extensive philosophical speculation and rumination before developing a specific obsessional problem.

In the seventeenth-century autobiography of John Bunyan, *Grace Abounding to the Chief of Sinners*, there is a 'textbook case' of intrusive thoughts of a religious nature:

'But it was neither my dislike of the thought nor yet any desire and endeavour to resist it that in the least did shake or abate the continuation or force of strength thereof; for it did alwayes, in almost whatever I thought, intermix itself therewith, in such sort that I could neither eat my food, stoop for a pin, chop a stick, or cast mine eyes to look on this or that, but still the temptation would come, Sell Christ for this, or sell Christ for that; sell him, sell him.'

Sometimes Bunyan was assailed with fears about future damnation, and at other times hair-splitting existential dilemmas troubled him. The inner words 'Sell Christ' tormented him. The following quotation from his autobiography suggests that at other times the intrusive images were of a visual kind:

'Also when, because I have had wandering thoughts in the time of this duty, I have laboured to compose my mind and fix it upon God; then, with great force, hath the Tempter laboured to distract me and confound me, and to turn away my mind, by presenting to my heart and fancy the form of a Bush, a Bull, a Besom, or the like, as if I should pray to those . . .'

Sexual and violent themes

Sexual themes for intrusions include seeing oneself, or those near to one, being in a perverse sexual role, such as committing rape. Violent themes, taken in the broadest sense of the word, include the thought of assaulting someone, being contaminated with cancerous material or simply watching a coffin containing mutilated bodies. Again, compounded sacred and profane thoughts of a kind can appear here. For example, Janet treated five Parisian mothers who were tormented by thoughts of damaging their babies with a sharp knife.

Sometimes it could seem that a person is tortured by unwelcome thoughts that lead to neither actual behaviour nor a hidden neutralising thought. Examples include the thought 'Christ was a bastard' or the image of mutilated corpses or decomposing fetuses. However, the existence of a category often described as 'pure obsessional' or 'pure ruminator' is disputed by the American OCD expert Fred Penzel in his book *Obsessive-Compulsive Disorders*. He claims that no one would be subject to bombardment by obsessive thoughts without taking action of some sort. The action would either be in the form of behaviour or at least an active search for some neutralising thoughts. Penzel describes these defences as 'compulsions', whether compulsive behaviour or compulsive mental effort.

Profound to trivial themes

Obsessional ruminations can be found at either extreme on a scale running from profound to trivial. Most normal, non-obsessional people almost by definition are able to avoid both extremes for either all or most of the time. Obsessionals worry unduly about, for example, why an apparently omniscient God allows evil (in the obsessive style of Woody Allen), whether the world has existed for ever or how many strokes of a toothbrush are required to clean the third tooth on the left-hand side. They might be concerned about the possibility of life after death or whether a discarded milk bottle top has been left lying in the High Street. The content of most normal thoughts has more to do with realistic and useful (purposive) activities – have I enough money for the children's holiday? There is, at least in principle if not in practice, a solution to such problems.

Depersonalisation

The obsessional thought can sometimes be one of 'depersonalisation'. The person is troubled by the thought that he has lost his personality, that in some sense he is not 'himself'. The *Journal Intime* of the Swiss writer Henri-Frédéric Amiel reveals such a feeling:

> 'Life is merely the dream of a shadow; I felt this with new intensity this evening. I perceive myself only as a fugitive appearance, like the impalpable rainbow that for a moment floats over the spray, in the fearful cascade of being that falls incessantly into the abyss of the days. Thus everything seems to me a chimera, a mist, a phantom, nothingness, my own individuality included.'

Neutralising thoughts

An intruding thought is usually (if not always) countered by a neutralising thought that seems to help to reduce its negative impact. For example, a thought such as 'the devil is good' might be countered by 'I remain a Christian'. The obsessional thought 'God is mad' might be countered by the thought 'I remain a Catholic'. Such a neutralising thought might serve very temporarily to lower the anxiety level of some obsessive compulsive people.

Some obsessionals accompany the neutralising thought with a simple action that seems to drive home the resistance. A good example of this was given by John Bunyan in his autobiography:

'This temptation did put me to such scares lest I should at sometimes, I say, consent thereto, and to be overcome therewith, that by the very force of my mind in labouring to gainsay and resist this wickedness my very Body also would be put into action or motion, by way of pushing or thrusting with my hands or elbows; still answering, as fast as the destroyer said, Sell him; I will not, I will not, I will not, I will not.'

Obsessions and compulsive behaviour

The nature of the link

The relation between obsessions, urges and compulsions can be illustrated by considering a 20-year-old student, described by Isaac Marks. He experienced the frequent intrusion of the painful thought and image that his parents were in imminent danger of sexual assault. The intrusion was usually associated with the urge to protect them from this threat. To do this, the student engaged in rituals of hand-washing. Although he admitted to the irrationality of his behaviour, he had little ability to resist it.

Another example concerns a 47-year-old married woman. For 36 years she had had obsessional thoughts and the associated compulsive rituals of repetitive behaviour, such as walking up and down stairs. The obsessions were first of swear words but later developed a sexual theme. Her extreme anxiety could be allayed by performing the ritual.

A distinction can be illustrated by considering another patient, a young data analyst. The problem, as she described it, was one of 'mental paralysis'. This was caused by repetitive and disturbing thoughts concerning something that happened when she was a child. An old woman whom she occasionally visited had died suddenly, and the patient was tortured by the thought that in some mysterious way she had killed the old woman. These thoughts had no accompanying urges to do anything. However, this same patient was also troubled by urges to expose herself when confronting a group of men. Like most such cases, the urges were resisted. It is interesting that, from what the patient reported, there was no accompanying obsessional idea immediately before each such urge.

Goal of behaviour

Another patient had been very seriously disabled by a fear of cancer. In order to counter this threat, she went to inordinate lengths in washing herself. Her hands were cleaned and disinfected hundreds of times each day, during the course of which the skin of her hands would be damaged and her washing water would be bloody. Still the ritual persisted. This example illustrates the important point that compulsive behaviour is often directed towards attainment of a goal or purpose such as cleanliness, so it can be described as 'goal-directed'. The goal might be perfectly normal, such as to get clean hands; it is just the effort expended to reach the goal that is abnormal. Similarly, the compulsive checker has the goal of, for example, preventing harm in the house.

In other cases, the end-point might seem bizarre or unattainable. There are situations in which the behaviour itself – the 'ritual' – might seem to be the end-point: an elaborate sequence of particular body movements must be performed. For instance, a person might need to turn around in the street exactly five times, or touch a post three times. In cases like this, though, anxiety might be reduced or the person might well believe that some future unwanted event has been warded off by the behaviour.

Disruption

Some obsessionals manage to lead amazingly normal lives in spite of what would seem to most people to be an utterly crippling burden. For example, a spell of four or more hours spent in the bathroom each morning can sometimes be integrated into the daily routine and the person might still manage to lead a successful professional life. Not surprisingly, obsessive compulsive behaviour often disrupts the person's sexual life, particularly where the obsession concerns contamination from others. Nevertheless, many people with very serious compulsive disorders still manage to engage in full and vigorous sexual behaviour.

Some common associations

The most common type of obsession seems to involve three stages:

1. obsessional thought,

2. urge/compulsion,

3. ritual.

For example, the person might be plagued with the thought that their body has been contaminated. This would be associated with the urge/compulsion to wash or take a shower. Given the availability of washing facilities, an extensive washing ritual, sometimes lasting hours, would follow. The three stages – the 'triad' – though abnormally and grossly exaggerated in terms of behaviour, might none the less be felt to have some essential logic.

Other triads would seem, to the non-obsessional, to have no possible logic. For example, a person living in London might feel compelled to wash his hands in order to protect an uncle living in Edinburgh.

Finally, it is possible for someone to perform ritualistic behaviour without having experienced obsessional thoughts. A person might simply take hours to get dressed, finding it quite impossible to speed up. The behaviour is ritualistic with a fixed order of doing things. However, there is relatively little or no fear of what might happen if the action is not done correctly.

Suppose that I believe it makes good sense?

Obsessive compulsive problems are particularly difficult to treat if people feel that their fears are realistic, a situation called 'over-valued ideation'. Dr Edna Foa described a particularly difficult and tragic case of this kind. Judy was a 37-year-old artist, with three children aged 8, 6 and 3 years. Her specific fear was of transmitting leukaemia germs to her husband and children. The following is an extract from the first interview with her:

Therapist: I understand that you need to wash excessively every time you are in contact, direct or indirect, with leukaemia.

Judy: Yes, like the other day I was sitting in the beauty parlour, and I heard the woman who sat next to me telling this other woman that she had just come back from the children's hospital where she had visited her grandson who had leukaemia. I immediately left; I registered in a hotel and washed for three days.

Therapist: What do you think would have happened if you did not wash?

Judy: My children and my husband would get leukaemia and die.

Therapist: Would you die too?

Judy: No, because I am immune; but they are particularly susceptible to these germs.

Therapist: Do you really think people get leukaemia through germs?

Judy: I have talked with several specialists about it. They all tried to assure me that there are no leukaemia germs, but medicine is not that advanced . . .

Linking the experience to gaining understanding

There have, broadly speaking, been two main approaches to the study of obsessional phenomena: considering either the *form* or the *content* of the experience. Psychoanalysts have been most concerned with interpreting the content of the experience, probing for a so-called deeper and symbolic significance. Graham Reed's approach, by contrast, is to examine the form, noting that virtually anything, from one's own death to tiny morsels of dog excrement on the lawn, can constitute the content of the thought. In this respect Reed follows in the tradition of Pierre Janet. Arguing that the content is too varied to form the basis for understanding and therapy, Reed instead asks such questions as:

• How does it feel to be subject to obsessional intrusions?

• How powerful do you perceive them to be?

• In what circumstances do the thoughts become most insistent?

By probing the form rather than the content of obsessions, Reed feels that we can develop models with explanatory power. Our own approach has been very much influenced by the outlook of Janet and Reed. This theme will be developed later.

12

Overlap and confusion with other conditions

A number of behavioural phenomena and psychiatric disorders – for example, depression, phobias and morbid preoccupations (this last is discussed later in the chapter) – have important features in common with obsessive compulsive disorder (OCD). And some so-called normal rituals are similar in important ways to OCD. It is useful to distinguish between the types of disorders but, over a period of time, a particular person might move around between them or experience a combination of several at the same time. The science and treatment of behaviour rarely work with neat, watertight boundaries. Nevertheless, trying to define some differences can be valuable in understanding exactly what OCD is.

Rituals and premonitions

Humans try to make changes in both this world and the next by performing rituals. In an article published in 1938, Sir Aubrey Lewis commented that obsessionals could be said to live in a world peopled by demons – of dirt, decay, death, cruelty and murder – and that they try to ward off these demons by ceremonies and rituals. Actions related to superstition have something in common with obsessional ones.

More recently, Arthur Guirdham noted the obsessional's: '. . . atoning and self-punishing symptoms which so resemble those of the ritualistic religions'.

It can be extremely difficult for an obsessional to tell the difference between a premonition and an obsession but, strictly speaking, the two states of mind are different. With a premonition the person feels that something bad is going to happen; with an obsession the person feels that it might happen if he or she does not perform a particular ritual. The difficulty for obsessionals is in deciding whether they are dealing with a premonition or an obsession.

The subject of rituals forms the crux of one line of argument on obsessional disorder. Rituals include throwing spilt salt over the shoulder as a means of preventing bad luck, rain-making dances and complex sequences of public prayer and devotion. These are performed in order to cause a desired future consequence (e.g. rainfall or the admission of a soul to heaven) or to avoid a future negative consequence (e.g. bad luck or eternal damnation). What labels such activities as rituals is that the behaviour has no rational justification. However, although we appreciate this argument, trying to decide what *is* or *is not* rational raises tortuously complex questions.

The rituals of primitive tribes seem to be connected with situations of personal danger and threat over which they otherwise have little or no control, such as drought, death, illness and childbirth. In general, rituals are more evident in children and primitive tribes, who have relatively few other means of achieving some control over their environment. Non-believers are more likely to turn to religious rituals when they find themselves in a situation over which they have no control, such as being in a storm at sea or on a battlefield. They feel helpless. It can be argued that the rituals do not change the course of events but ritualisers might not see it that way. It might, however, ease their anxiety. In their own eyes and the eyes of any others present, it might help to confirm the ritualisers as a member of the community of concerned and deserving individuals.

Touching wood occasionally, going to church three times on Sunday, making the sign of the cross in the heat of battle or performing tribal rain-dances do not, of course, make one a candidate to visit a psychiatrist.

Obsessional and non-obsessional rituals

So what is meant by '*obsessional* rituals'? There are three important differences between obsessional and non-obsessional rituals:

- The obsessional often repeats the activity many times, whereas the non-obsessional tends to run through a given sequence once. (However, this distinction is not an absolute one!)

- The performance of obsessional rituals often fails to reduce the person's level of anxiety – the anxiety level is sometimes even increased. By contrast, non-obsessional rituals seem to decrease anxiety.

- Normal rituals usually appear in situations of unambiguous threat, such as drought, epidemic or war. They also occur in situations of *anticipated* serious threat, such as displeasing God or condemnation to hell-fire. The obsessional is often concerned with situations that seem highly improbable, such as whether cancer can be contracted by touching door handles, or trivial, such as whether a row of figures really add up. Sometimes the concern is with something that most people would consider both highly improbable and trivial. (Again, though, we should consider this third distinction to be a generalisation and approximation, rather than absolute.)

Occasionally, for devout individuals, obsessional disorder becomes locked into and forms an integral part of their traditional religious rituals. These rituals become grossly exaggerated. This is well known in both the Roman Catholic and the Jewish faiths. In both faiths, procedures are available for assisting therapy.

Morbid preoccupations

It is useful to distinguish between obsessional ruminations and morbid preoccupations. A *morbid preoccupation* is where the thought has a rational basis and concerns realistic problems or experiences that cause unhappiness. There is no inconsistency between the thought and the rest of the individual's personality and lifestyle. By contrast, *obsessional ruminations* concern thoughts that are at odds with the individual's personality and personal history. Morbid preoccupations do not evoke the resistance that is associated with obsessional ruminations. Mrs P's case, reported by Stanley Rachman, illustrates the meaning of morbid preoccupations.

Mrs P, a 45-year-old woman, had been healthy psychologically. She married a man much older than herself, who then gradually became physically and mentally ill. Looking after him imposed a terrible strain upon Mrs P, who carried on in full-time employment. Mr P's problems reached the stage where he had to be admitted to a geriatric ward. Mrs P then suffered severe depression, which forced her to be admitted to hospital. Worrying thoughts never left her: they concerned whether she would ever be able to care for her husband again, and whether she was wrong to have agreed to his admission to a geriatric ward. These thoughts were such that she was unable to concentrate on other tasks. Clearly, they had a rational basis in terms of the context of her life, and this would be called a 'morbid preoccupation'.

By contrast, the obsessional rumination bears little or no relation to the actual objective circumstances of the person's life. For example, Samuel Johnson (described in Chapter 17) was incredibly hard-working and productive but ruminated about his laziness.

Psychotic disorder – am I going mad?

Obsessional disorder is different from psychotic delusions. The person with psychotic delusions (e.g. schizophrenia) believes that he or she is being driven by mysterious forces from outside. Obsessional disorder does not lead to insanity, except in very rare cases. Obsessionals stay in touch with ordinary reality in areas of their life apart from the obsession. They know that the source of the thoughts is their own mind; they have insight into their condition and usually recognise that their behaviour is, at least in part, irrational. Schizophrenics would not normally regard their thoughts as senseless nor would they try to resist them. However, in the past many cases of obsessional disorder were misdiagnosed as schizophrenia, and this probably still occurs to some extent even today.

Only a very small percentage of obsessionals go on to develop schizophrenia, a percentage that is no higher than for other psychiatric patients. However, there is a grey area regarding religion – an area that is a minefield of problems. It is interesting that some figures in history (e.g. John Bunyan), who would now be termed 'obsessional', attributed their blasphemous ruminations to Satanic influences. Earlier dictionary definitions of obsessions spoke of being 'actuated by the devil'. Bunyan referred to being assaulted by the 'tempter' and, as a boy of nine, being afflicted in his sleep 'with the apprehensions of Devils, and wicked spirits'. Taking a swipe at psychoanalytic ideas, Stanley Rachman and Ray Hodgson noted that:

> 'Bearing in mind the blasphemous content of many obsessions, it must be said at the outset that attributing the cause of obsessions to the intrusions of the Devil is more immediately understandable than ascribing them to the vagaries of infant bowel training.'

Noting that relatively few obsessionals become schizophrenic, Sir Aubrey Lewis wrote:

'The surprising thing here is not that some obsessionals become obviously schizophrenic but that only a few do. It must be a very short step, one might suppose, from feeling that one must struggle against thoughts that are not one's own to believing that these thoughts are forced upon one by an external agency . . .'

Because obsessionals tend to be well-practised daydreamers, when bizarre thoughts arise, the obsessional might be particularly well equipped to identify their source. One can speculate that, prior to the illness, the obsessional has often had extensive experience as a skilled manipulator of strange mental images and of living with the fruits of a rich imagination. In this sense, the pathological obsessional thought might often fit into some sort of historical context.

Phobias

Similarities with and differences from OCD

Obsessive compulsive problems are similar in some important respects to phobias, and a large percentage of obsessive-compulsives have phobias as well. Although it is worth understanding the difference between the two conditions, there is a grey area where a particular neurotic disorder has features of both a phobia and an obsession. A phobia often relates to more-or-less distinct objects in the outside world, such as snakes or open spaces. The affected individual might go to great lengths to avoid contact with the object of the phobia but, once out of reach of it, can often more or less switch off. The object itself or approximations to it can form an obvious target for therapy.

By contrast, obsessionals usually carry their problem around with them, however much objective 'disconfirmation' of the need to worry is presented – for example, reassurance is given that their loved one is safe. The object of the obsessional's thought is usually intangible and invisible; for example, hidden germs or a concept 'What would have happened, if . . .?' or 'Was I responsible for the death of the old lady?' Some of Pierre Janet's patients were tormented by philosophical doubts of the kind 'Suppose there is no God?' and 'Suppose there is a force of evil at work?' Obsessions are to do with events rather than objects, and these events usually have personal relevance for the individual.

The similarity and difference between clear-cut cases of phobias and obsessions were richly discussed by Guidano and Liotte. They commented that obsessionals say they fear situations but they then create a problem by their extreme effort trying to avoid them, spending much time scanning their environment and monitoring their own actions and thoughts. They 'create' in their internal representation (i.e. their image) of the world the very situations that they are trying to avoid, even when these situations do not exist.

Phobias, OCD and 'obsessive phobias'

A phobia can sometimes take on features almost identical to obsessional disorder.

> Jane, a patient of Dr Isaac Marks, was a 20-year-old university student with a phobia about pigeons. In the street she needed to make detours to avoid seeing them, and they formed the content of her nightmares. Jane needed to check doors and windows at night to make sure that a pigeon could not enter her home.

Of the more common obsessive compulsive disorders, some washing rituals probably come closest to phobias. Indeed, aspects of the two conditions can seem to merge into one, and attempting to draw a clear distinction could be highly misleading. A fear of germs might lead someone to take active steps, such as washing, in which case we would call it 'obsessive compulsive disorder'. At other times, the person might simply keep away from perceived sources of contamination, behaviour that we might term 'phobic'. A fear of contamination can, for example, prevent phobic individuals from visiting towns associated with contamination or confine them to a room in the home.

Diagnosing a condition as obsessional or phobic can often depend crucially on the individual's report of the symptoms. For example, someone who is afraid of leaving his home could be diagnosed as agoraphobic (afraid of being in public places). However, this would be wrong if, in fact, the fear was specifically of what could happen to the home if he were not there to protect it.

In some cases it might seem that a phobic condition arises from an underlying obsessional disorder. Consider the following example, described by Dr Isaac Marks:

> A 32-year-old woman had been seen by 43 casualty departments of

different hospitals over a three-year period. At times her fear concerned an imagined cancer of the stomach, at other times a brain tumour and thrombosis. Every part of her body had been X-rayed but no abnormality was ever revealed. Each clean bill of health was greeted by, in her own words, the feeling of being 'rejuvenated – it's like having been condemned to death and given a reprieve'. Within a week, however, any such euphoria had subsided to the point where she was seeking a new hospital for another examination.

The obsessional content emerged clearly in her discussion with Dr Marks: 'I am terrified of the idea of dying; it's the end, the complete end, and the thought of rotting in the ground obsesses me – I can see the worms and maggots.'

For many obsessional problems, such as rumination on a hypothetical past event or an existential dilemma about sin, the distinction from phobias is clear. The ruminator is obsessed with some event that might have happened or might happen in the future, such as a rape or death. Similarly, the compulsive checker is not usually trying to avoid contact with a particular object. Rather, their motivation probably arises from the desire to avoid an unspecified but undesirable state of affairs that might occur in the future, such as a gas explosion or a break-in.

However, concerning the area of overlap, Isaac Marks, in his book *Living with Fear*, uses the expression 'obsessive phobia' to refer to the syndrome that has features of both phobia and obsession. He defines this as:

'An obsessive phobia is not a direct fear of a given object or situation, but rather of the results which are imagined to arise from it.'

Two of Dr Marks' patients illustrate clearly the distinction between an obsessive phobia and the more standard phobia.

A man feared contamination by dogs, and spent time trying to avoid contact with dog hair and any possible traces left by dogs. He resigned from his job when he found out that a dog might have been present once on another floor of the office block. He would engage in compulsive washing rituals following any such 'suggestion' of contamination. It is interesting that he would prefer to touch a dog with his hands rather than let it come into contact with his clothes, because he reckoned that his hands could be cleaned more easily than his clothes. It would be somewhat inaccurate to say that this man had a 'dog phobia'.

Another patient's obsession was that injury could result from small glass splinters that might be on her carpet but could not be seen. She was less afraid of splinters that she actually could find and remove by her own hand. The description 'broken-glass phobia', without further qualification, could prove highly misleading in, for example, psychotherapy. It was not broken glass as such that she feared but the consequences of hidden bits of glass.

Tourette's syndrome

OCD is different from Tourette's syndrome, although there are similarities and a significant percentage of patients have both. Some researchers speak of a genetically acquired tendency towards both. Tourette's syndrome (named after Gilles de la Tourette, the Paris neurologist who first described the disorder) is characterised by tics – repetitive actions usually described as involuntary, such as facial grimaces or jutting out a leg. Unlike the actions in OCD, these involve a specific part of the body and, in the mind of the individual, can lack an end-point or purpose. Although the repetitive checking or hand-washing of OCD might at one level be described as stereotyped (i.e. repetitive), they need not consist of the repetition of simple acts. Rather, washing might be performed by using a variety of different movements. What is repetitive and stereotyped need not be the actions, but the elusive goal or end-point, to establish cleanliness. The individual's own perceptions are different in the two conditions, obsessional disorder having a 'whole person' frame of reference. The person with Tourette's syndrome is likely to report 'My arm twitches' whereas the obsessional is likely to report 'I have to move my arm'. The Tourette's person might be concerned because he utters obscenities in public, whereas the comparable obsessional would worry because he *might* utter them (but doesn't). However, the two conditions sometimes merge (as with Samuel Johnson, described in Chapter 17). The case history of a woman in Rome, reported by Guidano and Liotti, illustrates this:

Rita was 18 years old and single. She was brought to psychotherapy as a result of multiple tics and habit spasms. She had earlier been diagnosed as suffering from Tourette's syndrome. However, psychiatrists examining Rita at the clinic described the spasms as voluntary. By questioning Rita carefully, it was found that the spasms served to divert her attention from intrusive images of death and death-related themes. Rita was afraid that, if she were not able to cancel the images and they were able to persist in her consciousness, tragedy would befall her family. She experienced her compulsion as actively shaking the unacceptable thoughts out of her head; the muscular activity was felt to be correcting the weakness associated with the intrusive image.

Not uncommonly for obsessionals, Rita's thinking processes reveal an assumption of some omnipotence, of 'mind over matter'. An omnipotence, a kind of capacity for magical thinking, characterises quite a few obsessionals.

Not altogether surprisingly, Rita's boyfriend and parents did not understand the logic behind her behaviour, and tried to make her stop shaking her body. She was unable to explain her behaviour for the simple reason that to do so would involve uttering such unutterable words as 'death'. The attempts to make her stop served only to worsen the condition, creating a vicious circle. Rita's case is a good example of how interpersonal pressures can affect a disorder. Furthermore, Rita epitomises a way in which so many obsessionals see the world, and which might prove relevant to therapy.

Rita could not relax, even for an instant, with regard to the intrusive images; she must always watch out for them and never leave the slightest room for them. However bizarre the intrusive images may be, the problem-solving mechanisms in such people reveal rules based on their belief that perfection and certainty are possible in the relationship between human beings and reality.

Rita benefited from behaviour therapy. The treatment started with such words as 'death' being gently whispered in her presence, and progressively moved to where Rita was able to read aloud passages from books containing death-related themes. She was even able to walk in a graveyard accompanied by a therapist.

Anorexia nervosa and body appearance

Anorexia nervosa might be classed as a type of OCD. It overlaps considerably with disorders normally classed as obsessional, in terms of the people with the condition. It is sometimes felt that anorexia nervosa is a disease of modern times. Although it might be more frequent now, there is well-documented evidence that it has been around for a long time. Pierre Janet included it under the heading of obsessional disorder and treated a substantial number of anorexics. The feminist writer Susie Orbach in an interesting review, *Hunger Strike*, wrote of this disorder and conventional obsessive compulsive behaviour as ways for some people to cope with psychological pressures. They are ways of gaining some kind of control.

The anorexic person could be described as *obsessed* with attaining slimness or having a *phobic* avoidance of fatness. In anorexia nervosa there is the same perverse logic in terms of the difference between the anorexic's view of an aspect of reality and the consensus view, and the same resistance to rational persuasion. In both anorexics and obsessionals we often see a considerable amount of guilt. There is also an extreme exaggeration of reasonable goal-seeking, in this case to attain slimness. There is the dilemma of whether to eat, like the obsessional's decision whether to wash the hands. However, it is worth distinguishing the problem from more conventional obsessional disorders, if only because of the type of person who usually has anorexia nervosa – predominantly young women – and the specialised therapy techniques for this condition.

Sometimes a conventional obsessive compulsive behaviour gets woven into the lifestyle of the person with anorexia nervosa. Two examples come from Padmal de Silva. In one, the young woman insisted on leaving a particular segment of food on her plate uneaten, which of course reduced the amount she needed to eat. In another, eating was invariably followed by a complex exercise ritual, which burned off some calories. Anorexics treated by Janet used self-induced vomiting and had the same concern with exercise and the same paradoxical fascination with food that today's doctors and therapists report.

In this context, it is interesting that Janet also treated a number of people who were obsessed with shame about the appearance of various parts of their body. For example, someone with a normal nose might be tormented by the idea that it was too large. These days, the occasional woman seeking treatment for the size of her breasts might more usefully be treated as suffering from an obsessional thought. Also in his study of obsessionals, Janet included discussion of self-mutilation and hair-pulling. More recent publications include these as disorders closely associated with obsessional disorder.

Depression

Obsessions were once regarded as merely an aspect of depression, but now the condition is recognised in its own right. The person with 'pure OCD' does not have the more obvious signs associated with depression, such as loss of appetite and early-morning waking. However, obsessional disorder and depression have important features in common, and the drugs used to treat them are in some cases identical. Moreover, a significant number of people will experience both conditions, either simultaneously or in succession. Whereas 'pure' obsessionals will usually complain of being bombarded with thoughts that have at most only a weak link to their earlier experiences in life, people with depression are likely to focus on something more obviously central to their life, such as the loss of a partner or a feeling of worthlessness. People with depression sometimes feel suicidal – that they are both helpless and hopeless. By contrast, suicide among obsessionals is rare: even the most seriously tormented do not usually try to escape their torture this way. However, if the obsessional problem gives way to depression, the danger of suicide increases.

There is an important, but usually unrecognised, common feature in the two conditions: a feeling of helplessness. This is likely to be a helplessness with life in general for the depressive, but a helplessness related specifically to the intrusion for the obsessional. However, despite their feeling of helplessness, pure obsessionals often still manage to muster resistance.

Back in 1922, Arthur Guirdham noted that many people who seem to have no obvious cause to be depressed nevertheless exhibit self-crucifying characteristics that are similar to those of the obsessional personality. Such people were described then as having a tendency to 'melancholia' and to be characterised by being hard-working, self-critical, highly conscientious and exhibiting extremes of honesty and scrupulousness. This description is virtually identical to that of the obsessional personality.

We would prefer to see pure depression and pure obsessional disorder located at opposite ends of a continuum, with an area of overlap between.

| Pure OCD | Mixed symptoms | Pure depression |

At one end there are pure obsessions with no sign of depression. At the other end there is depression but not obsession; for example, the thoughts are ones that relate directly and logically to the person's lot in life. The area between the two extremes has features of both. At any one time, a particular person might be located at a specific point on this continuum, but could move around from nearer to one end or to the other over the course of their disorder. At any point on the continuum there will be negatively coloured thoughts, and the strength of the negative emotion can be increased by such things as stress.

Appetitive urges

Obsessive compulsive behaviour is distinct from what we would call 'extreme appetitive urges' or, as some might call them, 'appetitive compulsions'. This term means such things as apparently compulsive gambling, drug addiction and some forms of sexual activity. On close examination, though, the distinction can sometimes turn out to be more elusive than it seems at first.

In each case there can be an element of great conflict. Like handwashers, the heroin addict might admit that her habit is self-destructive but report that she is unable to give it up. If only she could break free from the cycle of injection and unpleasant withdrawal symptoms. The compulsive gambler is locked into a similar cycle that has an overall destructive effect on his life. In each case, as with OCD, there is a vicious circle and an outside observer often cannot see why the people don't stop.

Explaining behaviour

So much for the similarities; now for the differences. Appetitive urges involve what we would call 'incentives' or 'positive reinforcers'. An 'incentive' is an object such as food or a drug, the gain of which forms the end-point of a bit of behaviour. The term 'positive reinforcer' refers to the same food or drug and points to the capacity of its gain to strengthen behaviour leading to this. The person repeats the behaviour because of its consequences.

The unnatural agents heroin and cocaine act on the central nervous system like very powerful biological reinforcers such as food or sex. In a sense, they cheat the natural pleasure system by infiltrating and overwhelming it. The person in contact with positive reinforcers – sex, food, drugs and money – is therefore different from the obsessive-compulsive who is essentially trying to *escape from* or *avoid* a negative event, such as contamination or illness or any one of thousands of possible tragic events.

The excessive gambler derives pleasure in the casino although, as with all such excessive appetitive activities, the consequences can be painful. Such a person resists, if at all, because of these consequences. This reaction is in contrast to those of the obsessive-compulsive, who would be very unlikely to report deriving pleasure from hand-washing or the anticipation of it. At best the obsessional behaviour serves very temporarily to lower anxiety level, though even attaining this beneficial outcome is by no means assured.

In the obsessional's view of the world, the compulsive hand-washing might serve an obvious goal, such as turning contaminated hands into clean ones, or it could be in the service of a more abstract goal, such as preventing a tragedy from befalling a distant relative. This distinguishes OCD from an activity such as 'compulsive' sex, which is not (one assumes) performed with an ulterior motive. The pleasure of sex is itself the goal.

In trying to clarify the difference between true OCD and the condition we call 'extreme appetitive urge', a remark by Reed is very relevant. He said that compulsive behaviour seems never to be antisocial; the suggestion that child-molesting or fire-raising can be traced to irresistible compulsive urges comes better from defence lawyers than from doctors.

Another useful aid to understanding the distinction is to consider the type of therapy that is appropriate in each case: for obsessive compulsive disorder this is often exposure to the feared stimulus. The inappropriateness of this to appetitive urges such as heroin or gambling is obvious. A therapist would, of course, not treat gambling by exposure to a casino or child-molesting by exposure to images of children.

13

Who develops the disorder, and what is it like for them?

What kind of people develop obsessive compulsive disorder? Is there a typical sort of person? We shall try to outline some of the features that characterise the obsessive compulsive individual. However, as with all classifications, this process is fraught with difficulty – there are always important exceptions to any such generalisation.

People with obsessional disorders have often had what is known as an obsessional personality (described below) before the start of their troubles, but this is not always so. Also, having an obsessional personality will not inevitably lead to obsessive compulsive disorder. We need to be very careful on this point. People with obsessional neurosis usually have high levels of general anxiety and often low mood (bordering on, if not involving, depression).

Are they male or female?

Of the large sample of obsessional patients seen by Pierre Janet in late 19th-century France, women outnumbered men by over 2 to 1. These days, however, the ratio is about 1.5 to 1. Among compulsive checkers, men and women are represented roughly equally; compulsive cleaners, though, tend to be female more often than male.

Comparing different societies

OCD is not a recent phenomenon; it has been well documented over a long period. In early times, obsessive-compulsives were said to be possessed by demons. In European monasteries during the 16th century, techniques of *thought stopping* were employed. This technique consists of, for example, saying out loud or under one's breath 'Stop!' whenever the unwanted thought appears. Shakespeare wrote of the hand-washing compulsion of Lady Macbeth, and we have already considered Bunyan's intrusive thoughts. Although the general themes tend to be consistent, the specific content of obsessions changes somewhat over time, reflecting contemporary fears. For example, syphilis is now less common as an intrusive thought content, and AIDS is clearly emerging as a more common theme.

There is a remarkable similarity in the general themes that appear as the content of obsessions in Africa, Asia, Europe and North America. For example, among a population in Chandigarh, India, the dominant themes that emerged were dirt and contamination, aggression against oneself (including death), orderliness, sex and religion. There were doubts of the kind 'Did I lock the door?' A 41-year-old lawyer was obsessed by the notion of drinking from his inkwell. A 23-year-old student was bothered because she couldn't remove a current pop song from her consciousness. Interesting cultural variations on the general themes were also evident. For example, some people expressed doubts and fears concerning physical contact with beggars and people of lower caste. A study of Hong Kong Chinese, published by W H Lo in 1967, found a couple of people who feared penile shrinkage. This fear was attributed to the prevalence of such sexual themes in Chinese folk beliefs.

Padmal de Silva, who is Sri Lankan by origin, has documented the similarity between the descriptions and treatments for intrusive thoughts appearing in early Buddhist writings and those of modern behavioural psychology. Intrusive thoughts are clearly no modern middle-class Western phenomenon. They were around to trouble the unfortunate in the 5th century BC, for example, interrupting the meditations of Buddhist monks. Indeed, one Buddhist discourse is devoted entirely to techniques for controlling them.

What is obsessional personality? – a problem

There is an 'obsessional personality' (also known as 'compulsive' and 'anankastic') and its associated traits are listed below. One way to describe this personality type is in terms of the way a person answers a particular questionnaire designed to identify that personality. It is the widely recognised collection of a number of traits in an individual that identifies the obsessional personality. However, only a fraction of people with this personality type go on to develop obsessional illness. Similarly, a significant percentage of obsessional patients showed no sign of obsessional personality before their illness.

The relation between obsessional personality and obsessional disorder is a hotly debated one. Should obsessional disorder be seen as an extreme case of obsessional personality? Can we usefully see them lying on a continuum? Insight into the processes underlying obsessional personality might also shed light on obsessional disorder. We need to ask how the obsessional personality copes with the world, in the hope that we can see where things can go seriously wrong.

Some people think that the obsessional personality is fertile ground on which obsessional illness is easily able to grow. Others see the obsessional personality type as being like the property of brittleness of, say, glass (an analogy like that introduced earlier). Knowing about this property is like knowing that glass is more likely to break than flexible plastic when hit by a stone, but it does not mean that it is broken or that it necessarily will break.

What traits, attributes and abilities does the obsessional personality typically possess? Usually, obsessionals are found to have a higher than average intelligence. They tend to be more unstable/neurotic and more introverted than the general population.

It is vital not to assume that obsessional personality is synonymous with having an obsessional disorder. The package of personality traits (e.g. orderliness and cautiousness) that characterise the obsessional can add up to a person whose life is in harmony. Such an individual might well put their obsessional traits to good use. Careful checking and meticulous attention to detail can be an asset in, for example, editing a dictionary, making zoological classifications or composing a piece of music. By contrast, the obsessional problem acts against the goals, standards and self-image set by the affected person.

What characteristics comprise the obsessional personality?

People with an obsessional personality have certain typical characteristics. What follows is a summary of these – although not all people of this personality type need show all of them. Obsessionals have particular difficulty handling uncertainty; they need to feel sure of things and to have control. To be in control of themselves and their social and emotional relations with the world is a deeply felt need among obsessionals. They will study, measure and classify information, ideas and so on to try to ensure that, by being alert and using their intelligence and effort, they can control their world.

This personality type has a strong need to make decisions. However, perhaps paradoxically, rather than removing uncertainty by making a somewhat arbitrary choice, given the opportunity, they will postpone final decisions in the hope of gaining more information. For example, if given a choice of time for an appointment, obsessionals often have difficulty deciding which to accept, weighing up the pros and cons of each. Obsessionals are characterised by the desire for certainty, somewhat cruelly associated with the inability to attain it; the world of statistical chance is essentially an alien one. They have a tendency to ruminate 'What if ...?' The obsessional is indecisive – not having enough information available to make a totally correct decision, trying to take too many factors into account to be able to arrive at a decision.

Investigators commonly observe a tendency to perfectionism in obsessionals. They believe that an absolutely correct solution to human problems is possible, and this can give rise to awful dilemmas. The obsessional's indecisiveness represents an unwillingness to accept a provisional or 'working' solution and the need to scan for imperfections in any such solution. The virtues of alternative solutions are constantly weighed up in the interests of the perfect solution. Obsessionals tend to compare their actual performance with ideal standards, and to be strongly goaded by any disparity. Disparity is associated with tension and self-criticism. For example, in the past, when religious influence was stronger, obsessionals tended to compare their behaviour and thoughts with what was proper according to religious mores and dogma. Even in these somewhat secular times, a religious flavour is evident in the way that many obsessionals view the world.

Obsessionals tend to persist, not giving up until they are 'there', and 'there' usually means a score of 100 per cent. The craving for perfection is usually, of course, frustrated. Completion evades its pursuer. The dilemma felt by many obsessionals arises because it is impossible to please everyone.

The obsessional is typically always busy but never finished. In case you now feel unduly sorry for the obsessional, an optimistic streak should also be recorded: against all contradictory evidence, obsessionals commonly feel that tomorrow will be better than today, that the world will eventually yield to control.

Obsessionals often report a feeling of 'generalised tension': that something not done should be done. Some experts see this as a tendency to be hyperalert and watchful, ready for any problem that might be confronted in an often-hostile world. We might expect this to be associated with a frequent and inappropriate triggering of stress hormones. Obsessionals tend to experience what is called 'subjective discomfort'. This is not easy to define, but is not as strong a negative emotion as depression, and is by no means confined to obsessionals – it is distress with no obvious cause. Hans Eysenck referred to something very similar, if not identical, as 'free-floating anxiety'.

Obsessionals tend to be controlled, suppressing anger and outward display of emotion, and are prone to episodes of depression. Orderliness also emerges as a clear character trait, though there are exceptions to this, as a moment's glance at my (F.T.'s) office would prove! Indeed, the tendency seems to be for the obsessional's tidiness to be somewhat superficial. The desk of an obsessional might be very neat and clean, everything on it being arranged with great care, but the insides of the drawers are very different, their contents being crammed in, all in a jumble.

Obsessionals are generally cautious, reliable, thorough, precise, punctilious (particularly in the demands made upon others), conscientious, trustworthy, fair and well organised. Things are done methodically and systematically. They will try to impose a pattern upon objects and events. For example, it is probably more important to obsessionals than to others that pictures should hang straight. Obsessionals are disturbed by imbalance and asymmetry; for instance, some will insist that their feet should touch the floor at exactly the same time on rising in the morning. Obsessionals love to impose order on things; routines are valued, events are programmed in advance. Precision in the use of words also emerges as a trait. Filling in a form is carried out with meticulous attention to detail; recall of personal details is often performed with inordinate precision, and emphasis is placed on exact dates. Professor Reed has characterised this as a pedantic need to 'dot every i and cross every t'. Every factor needs to be taken into consideration, even those which by popular consensus would be seen as trivial, peripheral or irrelevant. The obsessional can suffer from 'not seeing the wood for the trees'. Such a person is an expert hair-splitter.

Researchers into obsession have observed an intolerance of ambiguity, which might be seen as an aspect of the need for precision. Plans need to cater for every possible contingency – leaving nothing to chance. The obsessional does not like loopholes, but loves clean-cut boundaries.

Obsessionals are single-minded in their pursuit of goals, with high levels of concentration. However, many also daydream a good deal.

When this personality type suffers from the corresponding disorder, there is an element of paradox: obsessions, which are by definition intrusions into the individual's overall setting of goals and aspirations, can coexist with otherwise excellent pursuit of goals. The obsessional will overcome obstacles to reach a goal, and the intrusions are just one more obstacle to be overcome. This personality type shows a preference for doing things one at a time, and doing them well. This ruthless single-mindedness can be a source of both awe and immense frustration to those living with obsessionals.

Obsessionals don't like putting things off to the last minute, and hate being caught without a plan and needing to improvise or make an impulsive decision. Nevertheless, they are often timid, sacrificing their own interests in preference to a fight. In his book *Brain Lock*, Dr Jeffrey Schwartz, who has treated over 1,000 OCD patients in Los Angeles, writes:

'I continue to enjoy doing research on the causes and treatment of OCD largely because people with OCD are very rewarding to work with. They're not only hard workers, in general, and very appreciative of help, but tend to be creative, sincere, and very intense.'

The picture of the obsessional painted by Arthur Guirdham is that of a misunderstood, self-sacrificing and tortured martyr standing firm on moral principles in an often hostile environment. The obsessional's heroic story as relayed to Guirdham was commonly 'I come to you with my troubles, doctor, but the people who come to me with theirs don't seem to realise that I have any.' Possibly Guirdham's own obsessional traits might have coloured his favourable perspective, and a somewhat less flattering portrait of the obsessional personality was painted by Alfred Adler in 1912: 'He is a person who feels that he is set apart from other individuals; who thinks only of himself; who is imbued with self-love, and has no interest in the general welfare.'

Except for Adler's opinion, it might be felt that the traits listed so far are by no means entirely undesirable ones, but there is also a somewhat more unattractive side to the obsessional character. Other traits include inflexibility, rigidity, obstinacy, irritability, moroseness and, perhaps somewhat at odds with the other traits, over-submissiveness.

Obsessionals are said to tend to be very careful with their money and to be abnormally anxious about their health, and some investigators have noticed a willingness to accept superstition. Our impression is that religious beliefs are rather commonly held by obsessionals. Some obsessionals report that their compulsive activities are attempts at repentance for their sins.

Dorothy Rowe's observations about superstition and the individual's view of what causes what in the world could help us to understand the basis of obsessional disorder. She found that obsessionals could not appreciate that their unspoken thoughts are private and have limited power. They had been taught that we can sin by thought alone – thinking murder is as evil as doing murder.

Some investigators identify two subgroups of obsessional personality, the one subgroup being people characterised by uncertainty, doubting and vacillation, whereas the others have the traits of inflexibility, irritability and stubbornness.

There is often fondness for collecting things. Time is precious to the 'typical' obsessional and is not something to be wasted on activities that lack a purpose. In this context of the importance of time, obsessionals often tend to be forceful and successful people who belong to the 'time is money' mode of thinking. Obsessionals are often masters of wit, by which means emotions are often tersely expressed. Samuel Johnson is a good example of this.

Among obsessionals there is a need to categorise into distinct groups, and to apply all-or-none logic. They tend to over-estimate the probability of harm. Obsessionals can seem to be unresponsive to rational debate. However, apart from obsessional personality traits – which, it must be repeated, are not always present – people with obsessional disorder tend to be very normal and with 'intact personalities'. The typical such person has been described by Stanley Rachman as being 'correct, upright and moral' and aspiring to 'high standards of personal conduct'.

Obsessionals like to abide by regulations and to be loyal to the institution with which they are associated. They tend to be conscientious and to conform to the moral rules, chains of command and standards of their society and to display a great sense (some might say an inflated sense) of responsibility. Indeed, Pierre Janet used the term *les scrupuleux* (the 'scrupulous ones') to describe obsessionals. Principles tend to be put before self-interest. Obsessionals often come across as self-righteous and demanding of others.

Although you will have noted considerable agreement as to the defining character traits of the obsessional, we must never be complacent. In case you are being lulled into feeling that the obsessional personality is well defined and consistent, another observation will shatter that calm. Some investigators have noted that, in direct contradiction to conventional morality, there are cases of what would be described as sexual perversion among obsessionals.

Moreover, some doctors and therapists have come to apparently opposite assessments of character traits of obsessionals. For example, obsessionals have variously been described as both immature and mature, self-deprecating and arrogant, as well as both timid and aggressive. There are several possible explanations for this. First, there could be ambivalence, 'bipolarity' or 'counter-personality' in a given individual. Obsessionals might swing from one extreme on a scale to another, depending on the context in which they find themselves. Also, as Graham Reed has pointed out, there could be just as much variation of some character traits between obsessional individuals as in non-obsessionals. Finally, different clinicians might be applying different assessment criteria. For example, Reed heard the promiscuous lifestyle of a female patient described as evidence of both 'loose morals' and 'an obsessive search for perfection'.

Obsessional disorder, crime and the law

It is very rare indeed (to the point of being unheard of) that an obsessional who ruminates about, for example, committing violence or an unacceptable sexual act actually puts it into practice. Obsessionals can often derive some comfort from knowing this. Pierre Janet studied numerous obsessionals haunted by thoughts of damaging their loved ones or committing suicide, and could not find a single example of their actually performing the act. Similarly, Graham Reed, after extensive study of obsessionals in Canada, could not recall a single case in which the antisocial behavioural content of an obsession had ever been put into practice.

Dr Jeffrey Schwartz of Los Angeles, who has extensive experience with OCD, was able to write:

> 'One thing that our patients at UCLA learn early is that, no matter how real their obsessive thoughts with dangerous content may seem, they will never act on them. No one ever does anything morally objectionable because of OCD.'

If the behaviour associated with the obsession causes only 'incidental' harm, the individual will continue with the behaviour. A good example of this is severe skin damage caused by extreme hand-washing. However, where the behaviour suggested by the obsessional thought would involve direct harm to the individual (e.g. suicide) or to another (e.g. stabbing a child), it will almost never be put into practice. In the overwhelming majority of cases, obsessionals do not come into conflict with the law. A very rare exception to this came to the attention of Barnsley magistrates in England in 1987. Prosecuting counsel, Mr Martin Lord, described the antisocial behaviour of a Mrs Y.

> 'She creeps up neighbours' driveways, or climbs over their fences, to peer through their windows, rummage through their dustbins, and peek through their letter boxes.'

Mrs Y's obsession had begun 18 years earlier when she was 34 years old. At one time her snooping took 90 per cent of her waking hours but had been reduced to 25 per cent. Neighbours had been driven to moving house and to exhaustion and the prospect of nervous breakdowns, the court was told. Defence counsel, Mr John Dearden argued:

> 'This is one of the most bizarre cases ever to come before the court. She checks everything in the house before going out but cannot control an urge to check the property of others.
>
> 'There is nothing the court can do to stop her urge. The only answer is for neighbours to ignore her.
>
> 'She has suffered from an obsessive compulsive neurosis for 18 years. The symptoms are that she goes round checking everything in the house – gas taps, water taps, windows and doors before going out.'

Mrs Y was bound over for two years in the sum of £100 after admitting that she caused a breach of the peace.

Occasionally, an obsessional will come into conflict with the law as an indirect rather than direct consequence of the disorder. For example, Isaac Marks wrote of a woman who washed her hands as much as a hundred times every day, occupying hours of time and making her skin bleed. Her salary was not sufficient to pay for the quantities of soap and disinfectants required by her behaviour. She was arrested for shoplifting, and the bizarre twist to the story was that, because of the wear on her fingers, it was impossible for the police to take any fingerprints. It is interesting that her perfectionism did not extend above the elbows – the rest of her body was left unwashed.

A perfectly innocent obsessional might sometimes come under suspicion as a result of his actions. For example, a motorist repeatedly checking a certain street for the victim of a car accident could well alert residents and police. In a case such as this it might be useful for the obsessional (or his doctor) to contact the local police and explain the situation (take this book along!).

In Britain in the late 1990s the term 'obsessional stalking' was common in the popular press. It was used to describe some high-profile cases of people who stalked celebrities and also people who made the life of some lesser-known figures (e.g. a jilted lover) hell by following their every move. Again, it must be emphasised that this is a very different phenomenon from what is being described here under the heading of 'obsession'.

Marriage and the family context

OCD can sometimes lock the whole family into distorted relationships of interdependence. So much so, that it can sometimes best be addressed in terms of a complex system involving the dynamics of all the members. For example, the obsessional uses the disorder as a kind of bargaining chip with which to extract favours or make threats. In this set-up, love is to be 'measured' in terms of the amount of sympathy and compliance shown. In some rare and extreme cases, family members are sometimes led even to serious thoughts of murdering the obsessional. Expert help could be needed in resolving such conflict.

Family problems caused by obsessional disorder can be quite horrendous. In some cases, the situation is possibly even worse for the other family members than for the obsessional. Some obsessionals are able to dominate their families completely with their rituals, to the extent that literally every action in the household revolves round their cleaning. The bathroom might be put out of bounds to other family members for hours on end each day. Consider the 28-year-old teacher who spent three hours each evening checking doors, gas taps and windows before going to bed. Or the 19-year-old clerk who needed four hours each evening to do the same task, only getting to bed at 3–4 a.m. From Los Angeles, Dr Jeffrey Schwartz reports the not uncommon case of other family members being driven to living in a tent in the garden to escape from the house.

Occasionally the obsessional seeks treatment because of pressure from other family members and against their own wishes. In one such instance Mrs X was accompanied to the initial consultation by a somewhat desperate and angry Mr X. Over a 20-year period, Mrs X had insisted that the family repeatedly move house in order to get away from their home's contamination. Each new house, it was supposed, would represent a clean break, but of course it didn't, and the unfortunate family again found themselves confined to the dining room in order not to contaminate the remainder of the house. At the interview it was very clear that the husband rather than the wife was seeking help, though it must be added that such cases are exceptional.

Obsessionals are commonly single or divorced or separated. To what extent this might be due to 'free choice' or to the difficulty for both the affected individual and the partner of living with the demands of the obsessional personality and disorder is almost impossible to say, if it is even a meaningful question. So-called full-time obsessionals are particularly prone to marital problems, as one might expect. The more covert or 'part-time' obsessionals are less prone to marital problems.

For some people, their obsessions seem to be directly related to marital problems. In some cases, clear improvement followed divorce. Marital therapy seemed useful to others.

Some disorders associated with the obsessional personality

Compared with the 'normal' person, someone with an obsessional personality is likely to develop obsessional disorder. However, there are other disorders that also seem to find the obsessional personality to be fertile ground. These include peptic ulcer, colitis, hypochondria, anorexia nervosa and phobias. Some writers on the subject of so-called psychosomatic disorders, particularly associate mucous colitis (the 'irritable bowel syndrome') with the obsessional personality. It might be expected that the condition would be able to set up a vicious circle with the obsessional thoughts. Sweating, faintness and palpitations are also sometimes experienced.

Obsessionals and the Puritan personality

It would be interesting to know whether Puritans are particularly prone to obsessional disorder. By the expression 'Puritan', we refer particularly to the faith that reached its fruition in 17th-century England and later in the USA. Typically, the Puritan is someone of uncompromising morality. As Monica Furlong remarked, in her study of John Bunyan, concerning such a personality:

'It is not so much that he does not see, and rue, the cost of standing out against established opinion or mass opinion, as that he feels he has no choice.'

Adjectives used to describe the 17th-century Puritan include honest, brave, conscientious, suspicious, efficient, self-analytical, melancholic, God-fearing, hardworking and dutiful. Well-represented qualities include thrift, punctuality, pedantry, tidiness, rationality and perseverance. To the Puritan, above all else, life is a journey towards a future goal. Joy and relaxation, if to be attained at all in this life or the next, are for the future. For the present, there is work that needs to be done. In the words of Monica Furlong:

'Work, being both practical and often far from enjoyable, was a natural sphere of Puritan activity. It supplied the continual spur, the kind of perpetual discomfort, with which the Puritan was most comfortable.'

The journey forward is a hard one, fraught with danger. The Puritan is like an athlete under gruelling training, always trying still harder. Even one slip on the hazardous journey could turn into a fall towards eternal damnation; perfectionist standards, total self-control and permanent vigilance against the devil are therefore demanded. Time is not something to be wasted on pleasurable but pointless activities, such as dancing. In meeting the demanding standards, extensive self-analysis combined with absolute truthfulness are needed.

The 17th-century Puritan and the present-day obsessional share a faith in perfectionism as a goal of behaviour. The Puritan, however, tended to believe that perfectionism was attainable only after a long struggle, and possibly only in the next life. Obsessionals, on the other hand, are inclined to feel that it is within earthly reach. Indeed, occasionally obsessionals believe they have already achieved perfection.

There are distinct Puritan traits in my (F.T.'s) own make-up. I still find it very hard to relax if someone around me is working. For example, on visiting my friend Helen's parents, I would find it quite impossible to sit and read in the presence of their cleaning lady. I felt most uncomfortable attending the office Christmas party (at Lancashire Polytechnic), because it was held in a room overlooking a road where people were going about their business. Time is of great importance to me, and needs to be put to productive use.

The obsessional personality, creativity and the famous

When people with obsessional personality can use their traits of orderliness and meticulousness, combined with persistence, to good use, the results can be extremely beneficial. Samuel Johnson and Charles Darwin are good examples. Their works reflect their personality: both made a virtue of collecting, organising, ordering and refining details. In his book *Daydreaming and Fantasy*, Jerome Singer argued that, at its most creative, the obsessional style is shown in the philosophical writings of Immanuel Kant, with its incredibly detailed logical structure and its call for the highest level of morality.

Singer's observation leads to a particularly challenging aspect of obsessionality: its possible association with creativity. Creativity is normally considered to require an ability to explore different and unusual ways of looking at the world, to develop new ideas and products. It would seem to call for flexibility and nonconformity, which would thus demand mental skills quite the opposite of the rigidity and concern with minute detail that characterise the obsessional. Looked at in these terms, we might suppose that having obsessional traits would be a major handicap, as much a burden to creativity as carrying a heavy lead weight hung round an athlete's neck during the high jump.

It is puzzling, therefore, that obsessionals are very well represented among the creative. Of those having obsessional symptoms and traits, there are the composers Rossini and Stravinsky, the diarist Amiel, the playwright Ibsen and the novelists Dickens and Proust. There are also poets, writers and essayists, Bunyan, Swift and Johnson. Obsessional traits were shown by Beethoven and by the philosophers Rousseau and Pascal. In Chapter 17 we discuss obsessionality in the writers Hans Christian Andersen and George Borrow, the philosopher and theologian Søren Kierkegaard and the film-maker Woody Allen. One might also offer the theologian Martin Luther, and we would tentatively suggest inclusion of the biographer James Boswell and the writer Thomas de Quincey as well as the musicians Brian Wilson and Karen Carpenter. Clear signs of obsessionality can be seen in the composer Eric Satie.

It is surprising to find obsessionals so well represented among creative people. However, in the light of the obsessional's preference for fixed order and pre-set rules, it is even more surprising to note that creative obsessionals include a significant number whose work formed a radical departure from the status quo; for example, Allen, Ibsen, Darwin and Stravinsky. (Dickens is described on the website.) In matters of worship and theology, Luther, Bunyan and Kierkegaard each posed a serious challenge to the established church. Samuel Johnson's creative writing served as a vehicle for advancing profound social change and justice, such as opposition to slavery and colonialism.

What could it be that creative obsessionals possess that overrides the qualities that do not lend themselves to creativity? We suggest that one such attribute is dogged perseverance, but we suspect that this is not enough. After discussing the obsessional's mode of handling information, we offer a suggestion of what else might contribute.

Certain obsessional ways of doing things, such as neatness, orderliness and routines, might be seen simply as setting the scene within which perfectionist creative talent can most efficiently flourish. Anthony Storr described the work environment of Rossini, Stravinsky and Ibsen in such terms. In keeping with the interpretation being advanced, here is an observation of Dr Jeffrey Schwartz in his book *Brain Lock*:

> 'One of the ironies of OCD is that it enables some people to function at a very high level because their attention to detail is so great. Years of practising OCD rituals appear to create skills that increase their powers of observation and memory in ways that can be highly adaptive.'

Occasionally the detailed content of obsessions might directly lend itself to literary or philosophical themes. Storr argued that reading *Gulliver's Travels* reveals something of the content of Swift's own obsessions. For example:

> '... during the first Year I could not endure my Wife or Children in my Presence, the very smell of them was intolerable; much less could I suffer them to eat in the same Room. To this Hour they dare not presume to touch my Bread, or drink out of the same Cup; neither was I ever able to let one of them take me by the hand.'

Coping with an obsessional person as a partner

It is worth adding a few words about the social interactions between obsessionals and non-obsessionals, quite apart from coping with the experience of obsessional disorder. Information on the obsessional personality can help to prevent misunderstandings. Obsessionals tend to be goal-orientated, purposive and planning in their actions. Producing gratuitous remarks does not come easily to them, and such remarks spoken by others are likely to be attributed a more profound significance. Anything that you say to an obsessional is likely to be seen in terms of a plan, a meaning for life. The obsessional might well ruminate over any 'throw-away' or casual remarks to find a serious meaning behind them. Obsessionals tend to intellectualise a great deal. We would imagine that, if the verbal and non-verbal signals are in conflict, the obsessional would tend to put more weight on the verbal signal than would a non-obsessional. For example, body language might say one thing but the opposite verbal message might be believed.

The obsessional sometimes has difficulty accepting that others are not obsessional, often judging their behaviour by his or her own standards. This can occasionally be seriously misleading. The obsessional often has an urge to reform a partner to match an ideal standard. Not surprisingly, the partner commonly resists the conversion process.

Obsessionals tend to tell their partners everything. Of course, whether this proves to be good or bad will depend to some extent upon the partner and what they are told!

Summary

Some people have an obsessional personality that is prone to develop an obsessional disorder. The disorder can make better sense if it is seen in the light of how the personality functions. Sometimes it is convenient to refer simply to 'the obsessional', meaning someone with both the personality type and some signs of disorder. However, two things complicate the picture: the disorder sometimes appears in a personality not characterised as obsessional, and certainly not every person with an obsessional personality develops an obsessional disorder.

In discussing how to treat this condition, it is the disorder and not the personality that is being targeted. The personality type is not one that is easy to reform. Indeed, most people of this kind probably feel that it is the rest of the world that needs changing! The disorder is quite another matter and the person desperately craves a cure.

14
Professional help

Nothing is certain in the treatment of mental and behavioural disorder. There is no magic cure, but in this chapter we shall do our best to give a fair assessment of the possibilities. You can derive some help simply from learning that help is available. Very many people with OCD refuse to acknowledge that others have the condition, firmly believing themselves to be the only person in the world so affected. Contrary to what you might feel, though, you will not be thought to be 'crazy' on revealing all to a doctor or psychiatrist.

Broadly speaking, there are three main types of treatment for obsessional disorder, some of which we have briefly described earlier. The type of treatment depends to some extent upon the theories that the therapist follows.

- First, there are the methods of behaviour therapy. One such is the *exposure technique*; for example, exposure to the repeated presentation of the spoken content of the obsession, as in a cassette recording of the obsession. 'Paradoxical intention' (discussed below) falls into the 'exposure' category.

- Secondly, there are techniques that try to reshape the person's thinking process; for example, cognitive psychotherapy (also discussed below).

- Thirdly, there is physical intervention with drugs (discussed in detail below), electric currents or even, in the most extreme cases, brain surgery.

In Britain, the GP would normally refer the person to a clinical psychologist for behavioural treatments. Drugs could be prescribed by the GP.

Behaviour therapy

The rationale

Using an ice skater as an example, suppose he breaks an arm while skating. We could argue that the first priority is to repair his broken arm. As secondary considerations, we might ask whether the skating-rink could be made safer or the skater taught to skate better. According to this perspective, the primary problem with an obsessive compulsive disorder or phobia is considered to be the abnormal *behaviour* itself (analogous to the broken arm). This is the behaviourist approach, sometimes called behaviour therapy. It is often said, in criticism of this approach, that it fails to address the problem underlying the behaviour. The behaviourist would answer that we have no evidence that there is anything of significance underlying it. Even if we agree that there might be an underlying problem (the skating rink/poor skating), behaviour therapy (mending the broken arm) is still seen as the appropriate tool.

The significance of the success of behaviour therapy in treating phobias and obsessive compulsive disorders is both practical and theoretical. Help is available without the lengthy and expensive procedures once employed. In these terms, the problem is seen to be the phobia or the obsession *itself*, rather than something lying behind it. Isaac Marks argued:

> 'There is no need to look for hidden origins to phobias and obsessions. They do not point to dark, unconscious secrets which have to be uncovered for treatment to succeed. The anxieties can be cleared by working on the assumption that the sufferer needs to get used to the situation which troubles him, without any need to reconstruct his personality.'

Methods

The treatment of phobias and obsessions by behaviour therapy is one of the success stories of clinical psychology. Where overt behaviour is involved, such therapy has brought relief to a very large number of patients. One such technique is *response prevention*: for example, the therapist might sit with the patient encouraging her or him not to make the response, such as hand-washing. Where a fear of some future consequence is involved, the technique of *behavioural modelling* has proved useful. Suppose a person is afraid of going into a shop in case he gets contaminated. Entry into a shop might be followed by extensive washing rituals. In such a case, the patient might be encouraged to visit a shop with the therapist, who would thereby demonstrate that no harm comes to people who visit shops.

Some of Isaac Marks' cases illustrate details of the techniques. Let's return to Jane, whose pigeon phobia was described in Chapter 12.

> Jane's treatment consisted of gradually bringing her into contact with the dreaded object, in spite of the obvious fear that this evoked. First, the therapist asked Jane to hang pictures of birds in her room. She was then instructed to purchase dummy birds and to get used to handling them. In her first session of therapy, she managed to handle a pigeon that was being held by the therapist. At the next session, she was able to accompany the therapist to a park where pigeons were feeding, even though she screamed when a bird came particularly near. The story had a happy ending: at the follow-up interview one year later, Jane reported that she was no longer afraid of pigeons.

The logic underlying treatment of an obsessive illness phobia is the same as that described for the pigeon phobia, but the form of the treatment is necessarily different. For example, someone with a cancer phobia needs to be exposed *in his mind* to an image of cancer within his own body. To do this, the therapist might ask the patient to imagine that he *has* cancer, has only six months to live and needs to settle important family business. The patient is asked to imagine that he has been shown an X-ray that reveals cancer, and told that, although this might at first seem unreal, the truth of the illness will hit him later. With therapy of this kind, the patient's family is instructed not to give reassurance (i.e. *not* to say 'No, you aren't') to his questions of the kind 'Am I really ill?' Such reassurance would normally bring temporary relief, but at the price of strengthening the disorder in the long term.

Treatment of OCD is similar to that for phobias but can be more lengthy and tortuous. The nature of obsessions is sometimes such that we cannot come to grips with them as easily as with phobias. There is often no feared *object* or *stimulus* out there that can form the target for exposure, unlike a phobia over a pigeon or an open space. Thus, Hans Eysenck once asked me (F.T.) 'How would you like to be shut up in a mortuary for a few hours surrounded by corpses?' To avoid conveying the wrong impression, I must add that Hans knew I was feeling relatively OK at the time and that I had a sense of humour. However, I suspect that this drastic intervention might not work, because, for someone with a death-related obsession, it would not tackle the personal frame of reference (i.e. it is the death of oneself or loved ones that is the essence – the existential dilemma).

Obsessions often take the form of a puzzle of the kind 'Did I . . .?', 'What if . . .?', 'Suppose if . . .?' However, in spite of the fact that obsessions are harder to 'grip' than phobias, a modification of the technique used with phobias has proved very helpful.

Consider another patient of Isaac Marks – Ann, a 23-year-old bank employee:

> Ann suffered from a variety of obsessional thoughts and associated compulsive behaviour with the general theme of harm coming to herself and, as a consequence, to her family. She worried about having become pregnant, in spite of being a virgin. Ann was afraid to visit the toilet after her boyfriend, in case she should 'catch' pregnancy. A wart on her finger was imagined to be cancerous and a source of infection to other members of her family. Objects were avoided because they might contaminate her with, as she saw it, 'cancer germs'. Electrical switches were checked very frequently. Ann washed her hands 125 times each day, getting through three bars of soap in the process.
>
> The treatment consisted of Ann first being given certain targets to achieve, such as being able to cook a meal for her parents without carrying out protective rituals. She was instructed to reduce gradually the number of times she washed her hands each day. Ann watched the nurse-therapist 'contaminate' herself by doing something that Ann would have been afraid to do. The logic was to expose Ann gradually to the feared situations in the hope that they would thereby slowly lose their fear-evoking potency. The family and Ann's boyfriend were involved with the programme. As an index of its success, after the 47th session Ann had reduced her consumption of soap to one bar every two weeks.

Paradoxical intention

Rationale

A technique that has been used with some success in treating obsessions is that of *paradoxical intention*. The idea is to expose the patient not just to the feared object or thought but to an extremely exaggerated version of it. A patient who is obsessed with the thought that he might commit a sexual assault in public is taken by the therapist to a public place and told to try to assault as many people as possible. He is typically quite unable to begin to do so, and often finds the notion ludicrous. Similarly, a stutterer is told to try hard to stutter as much as possible.

The therapy is attractive in part because of the essentially *paradoxical* nature of the obsessional phenomenon. The patient is tempted to do something quite against her better judgement or feels compelled to think a thought quite at odds with the rest of her lifestyle. As therapy, the patient is instructed to dwell on the thought, to expand on it and convince herself of its validity.

Application

Consider a 22-year-old man treated by this technique, reported by Lazarus in his book *Behaviour Therapy and Beyond*. On visiting a cinema, the man was obsessed with the idea that he might have started a fire in the toilet, and would need to get up repeatedly to inspect the toilet. He did this up to twenty times in the course of a film. The instructions to the patient were as follows. When the urge to check next intruded, he should imagine that a fire has indeed broken out. The entire men's room is ablaze. Soon the cinema is an inferno. The fire rages out of control throughout the entire city, while the unfortunate obsessional who is the cause of it all is still seated in the cinema. On his next visit to the cinema, the patient tried imagining this sequence. At first, he experienced acute panic, but this gave way to a calm feeling and a realisation of 'how ridiculous it was to keep checking'.

H O Gerz, an advocate of paradoxical intention who reported success in its use, observed that, because most people with OCD are perfectionists, the underlying theme must be 'Who wants to be perfect? I don't give a damn!' A man who had obsessive doubts about whether he really loved his wife was asked to adopt the attitude 'Who wants to love his wife?'

Is the world real?

Along similar lines was K Kocourek's treatment of a patient who was obsessed by the thought that the objects of the world might not be real.

Just before World War II, the man, a 41-year-old Munich lawyer, had read the work *Critique of Pure Reason* by the philosopher Immanuel Kant, and a sentence concerning the possibility of unreality '. . . was the truly decisive blow for me, all else had been only a prelude'. From then on, the lawyer was concerned to do everything '100 per cent' correct. The symptoms improved somewhat during his period of war service. However, they later got much worse and he was unable to work. The obsessive thought of unreality was attacked with 'paradoxical intention'; he was asked to practise the phrase 'Okay, so I live in an unreal world. The table here is not real, the doctors are not really here either . . .' This seemed to be successful.

Integration

Paradoxical intention is a good example of where ideas from different schools in psychology can sometimes be brought together. The unquestioned success of behaviour therapy, even when using only images of the dreaded object rather than real confrontation with it, depends on the patient's peculiarly human ability to create fantasy from verbal instruction. Applied to paradoxical intention, the patient should so exaggerate the situation, make it so absurd, that he or she is able to laugh at it. Therein lies the paradoxical intention. The prescription is paradoxical, but so is the disorder.

The Morita school of psychotherapy in Japan has ideas similar to paradoxical intention. In describing their methods, Takehisa Kora observed that even a small problem with the mind or body results in an over-sensitive reaction, exaggerating the illness. Students with a morbid fear of wandering thoughts expend more effort on preventing the wandering thoughts than on studying and they become trapped by their symptoms.

Cognitive therapy

Cognitive therapy – logical restructuring of thought – works by the therapist questioning critically the assumptions on which the patient seems to be operating. It was pioneered by A T Beck, G Emery and R L Greenberg primarily by working with people with depression. A similar strand of the development of this technique is termed *rational–emotive therapy*.

Cognitive therapy might be helpful to some people with obsessional disorder, where faulty all-or-none, 'black or white', logic tends to be the norm. One way in which the logic of obsessionals is sometimes faulty is their tendency to over-estimate the probability of negative outcomes, represented by 'if harm can happen, it will'. The psychologist establishes a rapport with the patient and then asks questions to try to ascertain the major principles on which he or she operates. Logic from which the disturbed mental state could derive support is unearthed and then challenged. Clearly, each patient is likely to have slightly different patterns of thought, so slightly different counter-thoughts are suggested. The patient's ideological and religious beliefs might play a role in what is the best counter-thought. This kind of information will emerge in discussion with the therapist.

To try to modify the obsessional's feeling of harm coming is one possible approach to therapy, though this would depend upon the nature of the intruding thought. An intelligent obsessional troubled by a fear of death is likely to resist any suggestion that, logically, it might not happen after all or will not occur for ages. Ruminators are sometimes secretive and suspicious, so the therapist might need to tread carefully and gently. Obsessionals often have multiple obsessions and to obtain access to all of them can require a lot of careful coaxing and confidence-building by the therapist. There is sometimes a *network* of related obsessions.

Cognitive therapy might very usefully target associated sources of stress that could be fuelling the obsessions, such as lack of self-esteem and difficult family problems.

Behaviour therapy and cognitive therapy compared

For obsessions without compulsive behaviour, it could well be worth first trying the technique of confronting *each* intrusion with the thought that the worst situation suggested by the intrusion does indeed, or will, prevail. This is the technique described earlier for someone who was obsessed by thoughts of cancer. She was asked to consider repeatedly the *worst* features and logical conclusions that followed from her obsession. This can be very tough, but it could prove helpful.

If this method of confrontation fails or if you feel more at home with reasoning, you can try the technique of cognitive therapy. You can see whether any subtle counter-thoughts help to ease the pain by undermining any 'logic' that is strengthening the obsession. To do this you might need to make notes of what you are doing. If a basic philosophical dilemma underlies the obsession, then, in the context of trying to alter the thought processes ('cognitive restructuring'), it *might* – and only 'might' – help to read works of philosophy, literature or theology that address the issue, see how others have faced it, feel part of a bigger community. Pierre Janet was occasionally able to help his patients by pointing to faulty theological reasoning underlying the problem. In this respect, he was a kind of 19th-century cognitive therapist.

You can also try to experiment with arguing against the thoughts. Get a friend to play devil's advocate by taking your position and you then argue against it. In this, as in other situations, play it by ear and note your reactions.

Let us consider a hypothetical obsessional, Jim. Jim had a religious upbringing. At the age of 25, Jim is assailed by the thought 'God is not good'. Jim might find that, by reading works of popular theology and talking to a priest, he can undermine his logic. He becomes convinced that his fears are groundless and the pain of the intrusions eases. He finds an environment of social support. Suppose, though, that he can't find any useful and convincing answers and the problem seems just as bad or even worse. He might try confrontation with the worst possible consequence of his fear. This might be that God is evil, or indifferent to suffering, or that there is no God at all. Every time he ruminates he could try thinking that the very worst situation of all does indeed prevail.

Caution

An attempt at cognitive restructuring might make matters worse, for at least two reasons. First, it might suggest, or reinforce, the notion that a solution exists to what in fact will prove to be an insoluble problem. Second, the quest might uncover additional information that reinforces the problem. John Bunyan experienced this, though in the end he seemed to find an acceptable solution. Bunyan prayed that the Lord would spare his wife from painful pangs, and when the pain lifted he took this to mean his prayer had been heard. However, rather than permanently comforting him, some 18 months later it served to strengthen his torment. The response to the prayer implied that God knew all that was happening in Bunyan's sinful mind. Henceforth the intrusion 'Let Christ go if He will' triggered the painful thought 'Now you may see that God doth know the most secret thoughts of the heart'.

Although cognitive therapy has a proven success, in some cases we are doubtful as to its potential. The obsessional is an expert thinker, even without the help of deliberate restructuring or a cognitive therapist. Trying to make sense of what is going on, to undermine its logic, to subvert it, is not something that we could strongly recommend in all cases. For the obsessional doubt of the kind 'Did I cause a road accident?' we would rate the chances of cognitive restructuring working as being low. In our view, simply confronting (in the imagination) the worst possible situation is likely to prove more effective.

As far as any rational restructuring is concerned, Graham Reed has summed up very convincingly the nature of one problem, as follows. Most psychotherapy techniques rely on the detailed examination of the contents of consciousness and attempting to interpret them. Such activity can be of little help and might be harmful, as it encourages the individual to be hair-splitting and self-questioning and to get into circular arguments that are the root of the disturbance – in fact, to practise the very activities that are causing distress.

Reed argues that techniques that try to persuade someone of the irrationality of their obsessional thought content can sometimes be problematic, because, almost by definition, the obsessional already acknowledges their irrationality. However, even bearing this caution in mind, these techniques are useful for some. A number of obsessionals, who have full insight and acknowledge the irrationality of their beliefs, still find the challenging of the irrationality to be helpful.

Some other ways of treating obsessions without compulsive behaviour

With *satiation training* the patient is asked to generate the obsessional thought and to hold it for about 15 minutes. A related technique, in which the therapist plays a more active role, is as follows. The patient is first relaxed and asked to close her or his eyes. The therapist then describes the content of the obsession and the patient is instructed not to avoid imagining any of the scenes. Consider, for example, someone whose obsessional thoughts consist of hitting out at a child. The therapist suggests scenes that cover the content of the obsession, no more or less. Thus, the patient is prompted to think about hitting out at the child, but the therapist does not provide details about the consequence of the assault, such as it being fatal or superficial. To do so would mean going beyond the content of the obsession. The pauses are very brief, designed to be only of sufficient length to allow the patient to record his level of anxiety. Usually, over the course of a one-hour therapist-guided session, there is a decrease in the anxiety level. This method seems to help some people, but by no means all.

Sometimes the content of the thought can be undermined by such a technique even though the thought occurs just as frequently after treatment – a lengthy and very realistic thought is reduced to a more vague and transient thought. For example, the thought of a knife being used repeatedly to slash at someone is slowly converted into a neutral object gliding through the air.

For large numbers of obsessionals, the unwanted thoughts have been found to concern harm, either to themselves or to others. Such patients, reporting for example a fear of killing someone or killing themselves, have been found to be relatively unassertive. This has suggested the possibility that the obsessions concerning harm were connected with unexpressed feelings of aggression. The suggestion has led some therapists to consider the possible value of assertiveness training in helping patients to handle their aggression better. Whether such training might help obsessionals who do not display an obvious lack of assertiveness remains to be seen.

Drugs

OCD is often classified as a type of anxiety. However, anti-anxiety drugs (anxiolytics; e.g. diazepam/Valium) are not effective in reducing its intensity. There is also an associated risk of addiction. Some experts argue that anxiety is *caused by* the condition, rather than being its *cause*.

Concerning drugs, the link is closer with depression than with anxiety. A number of antidepressants have a beneficial effect on obsessional illness in both adults and children. The first of these to be developed was clomipramine (Anafranil). Subsequently, the drugs fluoxetine (Prozac), fluvoxamine (Faverin), citalopram (Cipramil), sertraline (Lustral) and paroxetine (Seroxat) have proved to be of help in treating the condition, and one of these is now more often the first choice for OCD. (These are the names used in the UK; in some cases they have different names in the USA.)

Such drugs have a beneficial effect with both depressive and non-depressive obsessionals. People taking clomipramine have often reported that they still had the thoughts but were not bothered by them so much; they have other things to think about. Activities that had been interrupted by the illness can often be resumed, such as work and sports activities. This leads to a natural diminution of the problem. That the thoughts persist but are not so frightening is very much how I (F.T.) experienced the effect of clomipramine. It is also how some patients receiving brain surgery for chronic pain describe their experience. 'I can still feel it but it doesn't worry me so much'. These drugs are often very effective when combined with behaviour therapy.

The time between starting the drug and feeling any beneficial effect can often be frustratingly long – weeks or even months. Moreover, the full effect might take many weeks to manifest. Help and encouragement to persist may be needed, particularly if undesirable side-effects occur before any benefits. Another factor is that obsessionals do not always notice when the beneficial effects do appear.

Possible side-effects of clomipramine – weight gain, dry mouth, tiredness, excessive sweating, unsteady hands, drowsiness, problems with focusing the eyes, dizziness, constipation and difficulty in attaining orgasm – can sometimes be a problem. (This seems a daunting list but there is no reason to suppose that all or even most of them will appear.) It might be possible to find a low daily dose of clomipramine (e.g. 25 mg) that has a marked effect on weakening obsessional thoughts but only minimal side-effects. Stopping the clomipramine treatment can result in a relapse.

The other drugs listed above are also associated with some impairment of sexual performance but this is usually less than in the case of clomipramine. However, some nausea and insomnia can be associated with their use. Regarding the impairment of sexual function, a doctor can suggest a sequence of a brief 'drug holiday' during which the person stops taking the drug for a few days. This could be sufficient to lift side-effects without a loss of the beneficial anti-obsessional effect.

Some patients have a suspicion of drugs and a fear of taking them. For psychiatric problems, there is still a certain stigma attached to drugs. Patients wonder 'Could such medicine result in long-term harm?' A lot of testing has gone into the drugs currently prescribed for OCD and many patients have benefited from them. Provided that guidelines for prescription are followed, the dangers seem to be minimal. The side-effects listed on the document that accompanies them are only the *possible* ones. There is no reason to suppose that a given individual will experience all of them. Some people have no adverse effects at all. The chances are that the OCD could be much worse than the treatment.

Finally, the herbal treatment St John's wort can be bought over the counter (without a prescription) at health food shops in Britain. Some people have found it helpful in treating their OCD. Its action is similar to some of the prescribed drugs just mentioned, so any use should be brought to the attention of the doctor. St John's wort can also interact with other drugs – sometimes with dangerous effects – so its use should always be mentioned to the doctor or pharmacist.

Electroconvulsive therapy

Of all the techniques available for the treatment of mental illness, none evokes more fear and controversy in the general community than that of electroconvulsive therapy (ECT) and psychosurgery. The technique of ECT consists of first giving an anaesthetic and muscle relaxant and then passing an electric current through the patient's brain. ECT has not proved useful in obsessional disorder, except where the disorder is accompanied by very severe depression. In such a case, it is most useful to see the ECT as affecting the depression rather than the obsessional disorder itself. ECT should be distinguished from 'transcranial stimulation', which is emerging as a possible help for OCD (see the website for more information).

Psychosurgery

Psychosurgery consists of cutting parts of the brain or removing bits of the brain in an attempt to control the psychological disturbance. It is possible to envisage a rationale for psychosurgery for obsessional disorder that fits a contemporary understanding of the brain. Repetition of a thought suggests repetition of activity in circuits of nerve cells, and a well-placed cut might just break the circuit. These days, psychosurgery is used in only the most extreme cases that have proved resistant to less drastic interventions. Some authorities still consider it a viable procedure in such extreme cases. However, drugs and behaviour therapy offer a safer and more viable choice. A tragic case of psychosurgery (reported by N A Jenike, L Baer and W E Minichiello in 1986) concerned a woman who believed she was contaminated by things associated with death, such as cemeteries and coffins. So serious was this fear that she was living a hermit's existence, confined to her bed and being fed by her husband. She was offered a form of behaviour therapy involving confrontation with the feared objects. However, so great was her fear that she opted to undergo psychosurgery, which she saw as a lesser evil. The psychosurgery failed to relieve the situation and she then accepted behaviour therapy.

The case of Tom (reported by L Solyom, I M Turnbull and M A Wilensky in 1987) is also interesting:

> Tom, a 19-year-old, had had obsessions regarding contamination since he was 10. By the age of 15, checking and hand-washing had become insufferable problems. Tom attempted suicide twice, believing that the sacrifice of his life would appease God and restore family harmony. Things got worse, with Tom also acquiring a chanting ritual. One day he complained to his mother about how awful life had become, to which she replied 'Go and shoot yourself'. In utter desperation, he took a .22 calibre rifle, and pointed it into his mouth. Tom felt that to fire such a shot would somehow answer his problem, which, apparently, is exactly what it did, though not for any reason he could have anticipated.
>
> Tom was found alive, but with blood on his face. The bullet was lodged in his brain, having penetrated the left frontal lobe, for which Tom was given neurosurgery. From then on, and at a check-up two years later, Tom's obsessional problems were minimal.

Was it pure coincidence that Tom's self-inflicted 'psychosurgery' was associated with a dramatic recovery from obsessional disorder? We cannot say. Perhaps the stay in hospital at a safe distance from the insufferable stresses of family life could have been responsible. Perhaps the drama of 'hitting bottom' and the suicide attempt played a role. Perhaps the change in his mother in taking a more sympathetic view of Tom was responsible. All of these factors could have played a part, in addition to any possible effect of damage to the brain tissue.

Final word

In summary, we can say that, of all the techniques available, behaviour therapy offers the most hope. Such techniques are very effective where compulsive behaviour is involved, and for obsessions without associated behaviour some techniques work for some people in some situations. Paradoxical intention offers some hope. These techniques are quick, cheap and not too painful. In our view, a drug used in conjunction with such techniques could prove to be more effective than any other combination.

15
Self-help – what to do and what not to do

On their own initiative, people with an obsessional disorder and their families can achieve much by helping themselves or, conversely, make some fundamental errors. The advice that follows is offered in the hope that you will find at least some of it useful.

Even if your attempts to block the obsessional thoughts themselves are not successful, you might have some success with stopping the process of 'ruminating about ruminations'. Any ruminations about ruminations need to be constructive ones, involving the planning of new experiences and modes of social interaction. (In the last few pages of his book, Graham Reed gives examples of some mental exercises that might prove useful in changing the general way that you process information.)

You can note situations in which you feel particularly bad, and attempt to avoid them in the future. Note also any in which the obsessions seem to be less frequent or less intense and try to maximise such situations. Try to identify any 'dismissal tactics' – those courses of action that are good at getting away from the thoughts. You might find voluntary work, music, sport, debate or amateur dramatics to be your best dismissal tactic.

Self-applied behaviour therapy

Without trying to trivialise the situation and with full awareness of the difficulties, let us say: try to bring *as much effort as you can muster* to prevent yourself engaging in compulsive activities (i.e. counter-reactions to the obsessional intrusion). These compulsive activities might take the form of behaviour or pure thoughts. Even without a therapist you might achieve something. Try to set realistic goals for a gradual reduction in these counter-reactions and enlist the help of a friend or family. Compulsive behaviour might not be such obvious actions as hand-washing but more subtle things, such as searching the weekly TV guide for programmes that could bring reassurance. Mental tricks such as using your imagination in trying to find a resolution to the problem also need to be resisted. However, try to find a diversionary tactic rather than launching a head-on confrontation with the obsession. For example, the thought 'I have AIDS' might be countered by 'one never knows in this world'. The version of behaviour therapy called 'brain lock' (described shortly) could prove useful.

Keeping busy

In general, we can probably do no better than listen to the wisdom advanced by Samuel Johnson:

> 'The safe and general antidote against sorrow is employment.'

Or, perhaps more specifically, when the problem is one of obsessional thoughts:

> 'Imagination never takes such firm possession of the mind as when it is found empty and unoccupied.'

We can see the rationale for this in terms of the brain's limited processing capacity. The brain is less likely to switch into fantasy when it is heavily engaged, particularly where there is a strong element of *external pacing* (i.e. the events in the external world to which the obsessional responds), as in social interaction. (*How to Enjoy your Old Age* by B F Skinner offers the same advice.)

When Boswell consulted Johnson about his own unwanted thoughts, he was told:

> 'For the black fumes which arise in your mind, I can prescribe nothing but that you disperse them by honest business or innocent pleasure, and by reading, sometimes easy and sometimes serious. Change of place is useful . . .'

Johnson was emphatic (as was usually the case!) in his advice to Boswell on what not to do, and you might experiment here also:

> '. . . make it an invariable and obligatory law to yourself, never to mention your own mental diseases; if you are never to speak of them, you will think on them but little, and if you think little of them, they will molest you rarely.'

Alas, we must note that, in spite of his wisdom, Johnson seemed to be molested almost all of the time by unpleasant intrusions. In our view, whether it is beneficial for you to mention 'your own mental diseases' depends on why you mention them. Insight and help can often be gained from others. It might prove useful to know that you are not alone in your problem. However, you should avoid seeking pity.

We believe that keeping busy is a good idea. It would be good to establish practical and realistic goals. Being under a little pressure could be good news. A forced pacing of your day, with clear target times, might help. A delicate balance needs to be found between, on the one hand, the desirable situation of being under sufficient pressure to occupy your attention and generate and realise worthy goals and, on the other, the negative situation of being under stress. Each person needs to find a balance.

Brain lock

A technique in the tradition of behaviour therapy and pioneered by Dr Jeffrey Schwartz and colleagues at the University of California at Los Angeles is called *brain lock*. It is described in the book by that name, written by Dr Schwartz. The book is primarily directed to obsessions that are accompanied by compulsive behaviour but an adaptation of the technique might be tried in the case of obsessions without compulsive behaviour.

The technique is based on the fundamental premise that, in OCD, the brain has developed a fault in its working. Indeed, the Los Angeles team was instrumental in demonstrating the nature and location of this fault (described in Chapter 16). Dr Schwartz describes how an obsessional can use the book as a self-help guide. It is based also on the assumption that you cannot fight the obsessions head on. You cannot set out to stop them coming. Rather, a certain amount of stealth is required: you need to apply techniques at the level of what you do *following* the appearance of the obsessional thought. Dr Schwartz claims that if you use the right technique the thoughts will then diminish in frequency. For full details of the treatment, you should consult the book, but a summary of the main points can be given here.

The self-help treatment consists of applying four stages: relabel, reattribute, refocus and revalue.

Relabel

When an obsessive thought appears, relabel it as just this – an obsessive thought, a manifestation of a disorder. Stop trying to find a deeper significance to it. There is none. In a characteristically American way of expressing it, the thought is 'simply garbage'. Think about it in these terms and thereby do some mental work on it. Reflect on this new 'significance' of the thought in terms of its being garbage. The obsessional thought is not a manifestation of demonic spirits or a failure of personality. Think consciously, deliberately and in full awareness along these lines. Don't just recite a term such as 'garbage' in an automatic reflex-like way.

Reattribute

After having got used to relabelling the thought, then, in addition, reattribute its cause. Attribute it to what it really is – the product of a faulty brain (yes, based on scientific evidence), like a glitch in a computer or a gearbox in a car that has got stuck. For instance, think of parts of the brain overheating as they work abnormally hard.

Refocus

This stage is when you do something else other than engage in compulsive behaviour in response to the urge; for example, play music, read the newspaper or whatever seems attractive to you. If you find it very hard not to engage in the compulsive activity, wait a little time before performing it. Dr Schwartz notes that with an activity such as hair-pulling it is essential to have something else to do with your hands.

Suppose that your disorder is one of obsessions without compulsive behaviour. We would suggest that a compulsive mental activity following the obsessional thought might be comparable to compulsive behaviour. This activity would consist of an attempt to neutralise the thought. Corresponding to this stage, you might engage in some other mental activity. Try to think of some pleasant image and work on that. You are urged to keep a diary of the progress that you make; for example, 'I managed to wait five minutes today before washing. Tomorrow I will try for 10 minutes.'

Revalue

Take another look at OCD and reconsider it ('revise it') as a disorder of the brain. An expression that Dr Schwartz suggests is 'It's not me – it's my OCD'. Another help might be to express the thoughts as 'toxic waste'.

Learning to anticipate when the obsessional thoughts are likely to occur and being ready for them could help you to relabel them. Using medicinal drugs in conjunction with the brain lock technique can provide 'water wings' to help carry you through a difficult phase.

Dr Schwartz points out that if the OCD is accompanied by depression, as can be the case, medical help should be sought to deal with the depression.

Checking

My (F.T.'s) experiences might be of some use if you are caught up in the ritual of checking. It *might* help to try in some way to 'tag' your check unambiguously, so that later it can be made to stand out from the memories of previous checking experiences. Otherwise you are in a vicious circle, where each check increases the total number of checks, and makes it all the more difficult for the latest check to stand out.

Suppose that you telephone for a taxi and are locking the front door. You check the door and it is locked, but you check it again. Then the taxi arrives and you notice that, instead of the usual taxi driver, this time the driver is a Sikh in a turban. You go to give the door one last check. While you are doing this, say to yourself 'I'll call this check a *Sikh taxi-driver check*'. Then, on trying to recall the check in question when you are in the taxi, with luck it might stand out unambiguously from all other checks. In this way, *today's* check stands out as being a real event that you have indeed performed, not to be confused with earlier checks. For another example, try buying an evening paper and focus on a piece of the day's news while you perform your checking. Then, on reading, say, that today is Blair's birthday, you might tag today's check as a 'Blair birthday check'.

Another possible solution is to take an associate into your confidence, explain the problem and ask her or him to observe your check. However, your confederate must be firm and not get sucked into the ritual. It is not enough to simply try reassuring you in some general way such as, 'I am sure you did lock the door. You always do, so don't worry about it.' In giving help, people can be more sympathetic than perhaps the checker realises. However, the helper needs to exercise great care, and it is very important to fit in with any therapy that might be in use at the same time.

Exercise, getting out and keeping busy

We suggest that, if you have obsessions and/or depression, you try putting the following advice from Samuel Johnson to the test:

> '. . . how much happiness is gained, and how much misery escaped, by frequent and violent agitation of the body.'

In this context, Johnson would doubtless have given his approval to today's jogging and aerobics, the 18th-century equivalent for him being a brisk walk from Lichfield to Birmingham and back – 15–20 miles. George Borrow (discussed in Chapter 17) found a similar solution to the problem of melancholic and intrusive thoughts, as described in *Lavengro*:

> 'I have come from some distance . . . indeed I am walking for exercise, which I find as necessary to the mind as the body. I believe that by exercise people would escape much mental misery.'

In an interview in the *Sunday Times*, Woody Allen related his own somewhat similar experiences that offer the therapeutic combination of a certain amount of physical exertion and rich sensory stimulation:

> 'In every crisis in my life, the way I have responded is by immediately putting on my coat and walking the streets endlessly.'

It would seem that the streets of Manhattan have a beneficial effect on Allen that is similar to the one Samuel Johnson described for London: '. . . if there is not much happiness, there is, at least, such a diversity of good and evil, that slight vexations do not fix upon the heart'. At times of particularly acute mental agony, Johnson was known to spend all night walking the streets of London, his massive physique affording protection against the capital's numerous villains.

Some people seem to find creative 'obsessions' themselves a good distraction from obsessional problems. For example, Woody Allen is quoted as saying '. . . if one can arrange one's life so that one can obsess about small things, it keeps you from obsessing about the really big things'. In this case, the really big things are death, ageing and the passage of time. The small things are presumably film-making and acting.

In this context, rest and sedation might well be counter-productive. They could present you with a golden opportunity to ruminate.

If you are leading a hermit's life, you should get out and about, and note what happens. Try taking a package-tour holiday. Try energetic sport, such as badminton or aerobics. Social sports might be most useful, and better than solitary pursuits such as jogging on your own.

The company of others

Samuel Johnson recommended early rising (something he was not good at!) as a means of reclaiming imagination, but perhaps most important of all to him was the company of others. He wrote: 'Happiness is not found in self-contemplation; it is perceived only when it is reflected from another.' Nothing could be worse than being alone, or going back to an empty house. To Johnson what was needed was conversation, '. . . where there is no competition, no vanity, but a calm quiet interchange of sentiments'. Sir Joshua Reynolds told James Boswell 'He has often begged me to go home with him to prevent his being alone in the coach. Any company was better than none; by which he connected himself with many mean persons whose presence he could command.' Boswell felt that playing draughts would have had a beneficial effect on Johnson's mental state.

Prayer and religion

People with OCD commonly pray to get better. In the pioneering 'brain lock' technique of overcoming the disorder, Dr Jeffrey Schwartz suggests that people who pray should do so for help and strength in their attempts to combat it. Dr Schwartz notes that religious people often ask the questions 'Why me? What sin have I committed?' An understanding of OCD in terms of the brain going wrong (described in detail later) can help to resolve this – they have done nothing wrong.

There is even the occasional report of faith-healing working, though not surprisingly we lack controlled studies.

Buddhism and self-help

Buddhist teachings offer help for eliminating unwanted thoughts. Padmal de Silva has described a hierarchy of therapeutic methods: if the first fails to eliminate the intrusion, you move down the hierarchy until you find a suitable one. The first trick is to try to move to an incompatible thought; for example, an intrusion of hate would need to prompt a thought of kindness. If that fails, you should try considering the harmful consequences of the intrusion. Next, distraction must be employed – for example, recalling something or engaging in a task. Fourthly, you could try asking what is the cause of the thought, and finally, if all else fails, the command is to try to dominate the mind by, among other things, clenching the teeth and pressing the tongue hard against the palate. The last is like a strong person restraining a weaker one.

Another piece of advice found in Buddhist teaching, having clear parallels with contemporary therapy, is to concentrate on the unwanted thought – confront it, think about it, dwell on it. It should then lose its evil attraction; it might even disappear.

Effects of alcohol and drugs

We advise you most strongly to be very careful with alcohol consumption. Alcohol will most probably make the intrusions less frequent and less intense . . . for a while. As its effect wears off, it could well make them much worse for a long time. The danger is that you might associate the alcohol more closely with the good rather than the bad effects. It is highly unlikely that alcohol would have any net beneficial effect on this condition. Samuel Johnson was particularly careful in his advice on the use of alcohol (though, at times, having quite a reputation as a drinker). Unfortunately, 'souls . . . sometimes fly for relief to wine instead of exercise, and purchase temporary ease, by the hazard of the most dreadful consequences'.

Johnson experimented with opium as a means of obtaining bodily and mental peace, though this did not have the same negative connotations in the 18th as in the late 20th and early 21st centuries. We would be reluctant to advise it today! There is, however, the occasional report of hallucinogenic drugs having a beneficial effect.

There is disagreement as to whether obsessionals are more prone than 'normal' people to drug abuse. Undoubtedly, a number turn to illegal drugs in an attempt to find relief from the disorder.

Alternative/complementary medicine and techniques

You can try yoga and/or transcendental meditation, but you need to see how they suit you. In publications about alternative medicine, there is considerable discussion of unwanted thoughts. The amount of space devoted to it supports the idea that such thoughts are much more common than is usually supposed. Perhaps alternative medicine forms a more natural resort for the obsessional – 'I am not ill, it's only my thinking that is odd.' We have no evidence on the effectiveness of alternative medicine, but neither can we dismiss it. In Bach flower therapy, white chestnut (*Aesculus hippocastanum*) is recommended for unwanted thoughts.

Prevention and some warning signs

Can one do anything to prevent obsessional disorder? We can give some cautious advice to parents, care-givers and careers advisers etc. Be open with your child. Tell them truthfully about life and its problems, good and bad. Encourage a richness of experience. Answer their questions truthfully. Of course protect your child, but don't be over-protective. Don't 'wrap the child in cotton wool'. Try not to make the child feel superior or inferior to others.

Both in Britain and in Hong Kong it was observed that the parents of obsessional neurotics tended, more than average, to have strict perfectionist standards that were expected of their children. So the advice to parents would be to avoid setting rigid and perfectionist standards. Goals should be accessible. (Such advice is probably equally useful for avoiding depression.)

In 1987 Roger Pitman offered advice to parents of children who seem to have a predisposition towards obsessional disorder:

> 'One should mistrust wisdom, over-prudence and reflection in children. These children should be encouraged to confront reality and even be allowed to have dangerous experiences, which are exhilarating and increase self-confidence. They should be encouraged not to avoid fights with peers; concern about their futures is worth the risk of a few punches. The physical should be emphasised over the intellectual. They should not be given the chance to daydream, but pushed towards quickness, accuracy and practical activity. Unfortunately, the parents of these patients often do the opposite. Nothing makes a child timid like the presence of his parents, because in their presence he does not feel the need to make an effort.'

In our view, it is unreasonable to try to eliminate daydreaming. Rather, a reasonable balance between daydreaming and activity is desirable. Active sport with other people (e.g. aerobics) could prove to have a beneficial effect.

Jobs and career guidance

Our hunch (and we put it no stronger than that) is that, all else being equal, obsessionals probably do better, in terms of their peace of mind, by being in jobs that discourage too much independent free-thinking. However, the main criterion on career guidance is to avoid undue stress that would exacerbate the OCD, and obsessionals sometimes show a flair for creativity. They can be found in pursuit of a wide variety of careers. We suggest that, if there is a choice, they are steered towards jobs in which some kind of external pacing is involved and where there is limited time for free-floating thought. Possibly politics, social work, voluntary work, teaching, nursing or the probation service could make good careers. In 1938, Sir Aubrey Lewis offered the advice:

> '. . . it is usually better for an obsessional to have his day mapped out as far as possible, without frequent need of choosing between various courses of action; sub-editing a newspaper, for example, or speculating on the stock exchange are the reverse of ideal occupations for him.'

What can a partner or friend do to help?

Obsessions often involve not just the affected individual but also the family. The whole family might sometimes be usefully involved in the therapeutic process. In some cases other family members are being used or exploited to serve the compulsive behaviour. It is not unknown for obsessionals to use their condition in order to manipulate others. Sometimes family members could be described as acting in collusion with the obsessional. In extreme but rare cases, the obsessive compulsive will tyrannise other family members into submission, under threat of temper tantrums or physical abuse.

For the close companion of an obsessional neurotic, we offer some advice. However, if the obsessional person is undergoing treatment, it is vital that the therapist be contacted. What could seem to be help might in fact be going counter to the treatment. For example, to comply with an obsessional's wishes for reassurance, or for leaving the bathroom unoccupied all evening, could directly hinder therapy. Fundamental reorganisation of the household and its interpersonal relations might help to find a solution to the problem, such as lowering stress levels in the family. If the other family members are complying under duress or threat, clearly they are in a real dilemma. In *Living with Fear*, Isaac Marks says:

> 'Should they settle for a quiet life and just comply with the patient's weird requests to avoid upsetting him or her, or should they refuse and risk a flood of abuse pouring over them, not to mention the handicap to their own lives that will ensue? Gentle but firm refusal to comply is in fact kinder in the long run, despite the initial upset that this may cause.'

Occasionally, an obsessional has been put off seeking professional help by being laughed at by family members when making the first step of 'going public'. The necessity to avoid this is, of course, obvious. Try to be as sympathetic as possible, but be careful to give practical help rather than pity. Pity might help to confirm the obsessional's fears that he or she is a most unfortunate soul to be suffering in this exceptional way, and could make them feel on the slippery slope to insanity. Undramatic, genuine sympathy and practical help are needed. If it seems appropriate, you might point out that relatively few obsessionals end up in mental hospitals and that all but the most severe cases are able to carry on working. (However, if the main theme of the obsession itself is a fear of insanity, it could be advisable to avoid responding to pleas for reassurance. Such reassurance could run counter to the need to expose the obsessional to their fear, which might be part of ongoing therapy.) In his book *The Doctor and the Soul*, Viktor Frankl distinguishes between the fear that the content of the obsession arouses and fear of the obsession itself. It would seem that the situation is exacerbated by the person's fear of the obsession itself – that it might lead to insanity or suicide. Frankl believes that overcoming fear of the obsession can set the scene for tackling the content. It is at this level, of breaking the vicious circle, that paradoxical intention (see Chapter 14) enters the picture. There is not a high risk of obsessionals killing others or themselves.

Almost all people experience intrusive thoughts of an unacceptable nature at some time in their lives. Obsessional disorder is an exaggeration of this. You are not evil or being possessed by a spirit, but simply someone whose way of processing information has gone wrong. You are not being punished for your sins.

Your partner as well as you might need to face the fact that stresses and tensions in the family could either have triggered the disorder or are making it worse. There might be practical steps that can be taken to reduce conflict and stress levels in the family, and we urge you very strongly to follow them. Marriage guidance counselling and family therapy could well be useful. The family can often work as a team to correct what has gone wrong. You can all try to agree to target goals (e.g. a gradual percentage reduction in time spent washing) and a system of rewards (sometimes given the behavioural psychology term 'positive reinforcement') agreed for attaining each successive goal. Praise can serve as an effective reward. Consent and trust are very important. In their desperation, other family members are sometimes tempted to try radical 'exposure therapy', such as surreptitiously switching off the water at the main supply while the obsessional washes. This is very likely to make the condition worse and is a temptation to be resisted. An unpleasant 'scene' is a likely outcome. A system that has been used very effectively in the USA consists of what is termed a *multifamily psychoeducational support group*. In this programme several families meet together with a professional and set up a mutual support network, involving, for example, internet or telephone contact. They can encourage each other, offer practical tips and reward success.

We advise the avoidance of homespun psychoanalysis and 'trying to get to the root of the problem' of the obsessional phenomena themselves. Any restructuring of the obsessional's mental world that you might be tempted to try has probably been tried countless times already by that individual. Avoid at all costs advice of the kind 'You really must sort yourself out, otherwise you will ruin the rest of your life.' The obsessional needs no confirmation of that. Also avoid giving advice of the kind 'You must simply try harder to get rid of the thoughts. Make a really determined effort this weekend, for my sake' or 'Just stop washing, for your sake and mine'. A conscious effort to get rid of the thoughts, in the absence of any 'tricks of the trade' such as 'brain lock' or a strategy of confrontation with the worst consequences of the fear, is almost certainly doomed to failure. In fact, it is likely to exacerbate the condition. (Ruminators might even try to make no effort at all to oppose the intrusion but, perhaps with the help of their spouse or partner, set aside a period of time each day in order to ruminate *actively*, a kind of homework. Intrusions at other times could be answered by the counter-thought – 'We will think about this some more this evening in the homework period.')

Listen particularly carefully to the person's reports of what is good and bad for her or him. Obsessionals are usually articulate people who can describe their situation rather well. You could be of great help in, for example, planning ahead so as to avoid or prevent negative contexts such as situations of great stress. You might be invaluable in helping the person to get into favourable contexts; for example, travel or just getting out and about.

If compulsive checking is the problem, you might be in a position to offer significant help, but make sure that you really are lowering the obsessional's fear level on a long-term basis. You might be buying temporary peace at the price of worsening the condition in the longer term. For example, if you are tempted to accompany the checker on her or his rounds to confirm the check, this could strengthen the habit. On the other hand, to monitor progress as the obsessional tries to reduce the checking could be very useful. To make sure that you are not undoing the effects of any professional intervention, discuss all such issues with the therapist.

Believe the obsessional. Even if there are few outward signs of suffering, the person might be in considerable distress. Even when times were bad, I (F.T.) met people who found it very difficult to accept that I had any problem, simply because I seemed to be functioning normally. Obsessionals usually manage to carry on working normally, except in the most severe cases.

Walter Bate, in his biography of Samuel Johnson, discusses the subject of the relation of those with mental disorder to their companions:

> 'Only those who themselves have come close to mental breakdown – and not merely for a short while but for a period of some years – know how easy it is to disguise their situation from others unless living with them constantly (and even then it can be concealed to a surprising extent). Few people otherwise ever believe this is possible. It is too far from their own experience. But the truth is that most people, as Johnson often said, are far too preoccupied with their own problems, whether large or small, to pay close attention to those of others unless they are almost thrust into their faces.'

Finally, if therapy for compulsive behaviour is successful, a vacuum might be left in the life of the person. The six hours each day previously spent washing now need to be filled with something else. The more rewarding this something is, the less the chances of relapse. A partner could prove to be of invaluable assistance here. We wish you well.

16
Trying to solve the puzzle

Obsessions and compulsions are a profound challenge to psychology. Like other challenges, there is more than one logical starting point when attempting to make some sense out of them. For a start, we could ask whether it is useful to regard obsessions as an illness. Alternatively, are they to be seen as just a great exaggeration of normal thinking and behaviour? We cannot rule out the possibility that they have some useful function, though we imagine that we would need to stretch lateral thinking to breaking point to find one.

Is OCD an illness?

There are several related answers to this. Let's first take an unambiguous illness, AIDS, in order to draw a comparison. Here we see a clearly identified target in the cells of the body, and specifying the target gives unambiguous pointers to the kind of treatment that is necessary. The disease was acquired at a particular time and in a particular way, and to some extent one can predict the onset of symptoms. OCD is clearly rather different.

Consider an analogy between obsessional illness and alcoholism. The 'disease' label (or 'model') has not proved very fruitful in understanding the causes of alcoholism. Rather, it is more useful to look at alcoholism as an exaggeration of behaviour that most of us can handle without too much difficulty. However, there is more than one valid way to consider a given problem and the disease model was at least an improvement over its predecessors. Hitherto, alcoholism had been seen as the outcome of a weak will; essentially alcoholics needed to pull themselves together. Regarding it as a disease suggests sympathy and help.

Championing the idea that obsession and compulsion are diseases probably also has a subtle but profound influence on the people with the disorder. What is their own self-image like? Do they play the role of a sick person? To label a problem as an illness might be viewed as placing the responsibility for getting better firmly in the hands of the care-givers. Instead of actively resisting the problem, obsessionals and those around them could just accept it. For obsessive compulsive behaviour, the term 'emotional and behavioural problem' is preferable to a label of 'disease'. There is seldom a clear starting point for such a disorder, and the former term relates to the continuity of development and experience that in some cases will lead to the problem, which underlines the many factors involved. This prompts the question as to which factors promote and which discourage the emergence of the disorder.

Analogies can help us to understand what is going on. Suppose that the obsessional is like a computer that has been wrongly programmed and has got locked into a loop from which it cannot escape. Another approach is to ask 'Can we make sense of obsessive compulsive behaviour from the viewpoint of the theory of evolution?' That is, in what way is the evolution of the human brain such that it has reached a degree of complexity that makes the disorder likely? Such malfunction might represent the inevitable price some of us have to pay for the human species having the most sophisticated brain.

Such questions and any answers to them should not be thought to be mutually exclusive; it is in the best scientific traditions to attempt to tackle a problem in several different ways. The tentative answers will seem rather different according to the way that we approach the phenomenon. They will also depend on why we are asking the question and what is in it for us in giving a particular answer. For example, there might be certain advantages in regarding obsessions as an illness. In the interests of getting resources allocated for treatment, we might wish to emphasise the disease model, the suffering, the loss of working hours and the hope of bringing relief. On the other hand, the disease model might prove to be less useful in speculating as to the causes of the problem.

The disease model could be very useful if it serves to highlight the abnormalities of the brain that are a feature of OCD (described shortly). In such terms, the individual might be helped to view OCD as brain disorder and to stop seeing it as a sign of weakness or as something the deep significance of which needs to be sought.

Animals under stress – a suitable model?

One approach that psychologists have taken in trying to understand human behaviour has been to look at animal (i.e. non-human) behaviour. If, by studying the animal's behaviour (the 'model'), we can see similarities between the behaviour of animals and of humans, we might be able to cast some light on the more complex human situation. In several cases, animal studies have proved useful in giving insight into abnormal human behaviour – for example, in learning, obesity and anxiety.

Should we think of obsessions as a peculiarly human challenge, because so much of the evidence for their existence depends on spoken language? For the researcher into obsessions there might be no other source of evidence than the word of the obsessional. Although experimental behaviour testing in rats has so far not provided us with convincing insight into processes that underlie OCD, progress has been made. Also, clinical psychologists who treat OCD by behaviour therapy owe much to research using rats and dogs. For example, the response-prevention technique of trying to combat compulsions (described in Chapter 14) was inspired by studies with rats.

In people who have obsessions that are accompanied by bizarre compulsions of a ritualistic nature, it might be profitable to look at behaviour in domestic animals. There are cases where animal behaviour seems to have the qualities of the bizarre, exaggerated and being inappropriate, such as self-mutilation, though we need to be cautious in extrapolating to humans.

A situation in which abnormal behaviour comes into sharp relief is that of intensive farming. Some of these abnormalities might have more in common with the human phenomenon of tics, but they might also have relevance for compulsive behaviour. Veal calves raised in such a way that they cannot turn round and with minimal social contact display odd movements. One of the best known of these is 'tongue playing' in which the tongue is rolled in and out or swayed from side to side.

As a means of saving space, pregnant sows are often kept tethered. In this condition, the sows develop such behaviour as 'sham chewing' (making chewing movements though they have nothing in their mouths) and biting a bar of their pen. Group-housed pigs bite each other's tails, which can cause serious injury (in 1985 some 100,000 pigs were reported as being lost annually in the Netherlands, as a result). These behaviours are termed 'abnormal' because they do not occur if the animals are raised under more natural conditions. This is not far removed from humans who compulsively bite their fingernails or pull out their hair, disorders often associated with OCD. With all due respect to Samuel Johnson, we cannot help but think of behavioural abnormality in caged animals when we read James Boswell's account of Johnson's behaviour:

'In the intervals of articulating he made various sounds with his mouth, sometimes as if ruminating, or what is called chewing the cud, sometimes giving a half whistle, sometimes making his tongue play backwards from the roof of his mouth, as if clucking like a hen, and sometimes protruding it against his upper gums in front . . .'

It is possible that further examination of abnormalities in domestic animals and using lateral thinking will be able to enlighten us about OCD.

Does obsessional disorder serve a purpose?

If we consider compulsive behaviour in terms of Charles Darwin's theory of evolution, we might look for some advantage in the behaviour. In these terms, obsessions seem to be clearly 'maladaptive' – they act counter to the survival and reproduction chances of the individual. They break up the flow of purposive activity in which the individual is engaged, activity that is directed to practical goals. In the extreme, social bonds and families are torn apart.

However, from the perspective of a function served, obsessions can be seen as a pathological *exaggeration* of a perfectly useful process. When there is a threat it makes sense to focus our attention on it until resolution is found. In our evolution, threats would have been posed by such things as foul odours, floods, wild animals and rival tribes. Vigilance in the face of such danger would have put our ancestors at an advantage. We still have a brain that is equipped to look for danger and focus on it, and OCD could be the inevitable price that we pay for this.

Some writers of a psychoanalytic persuasion have suggested that, by emerging into consciousness, insistent and repetitive thoughts serve to distract the person from more unpleasant material that is also being processed in the brain. However, Salzman admitted that:

'The distracting or controlling function of such a thought is comparatively more difficult to recognise when the thought itself is extremely upsetting and disturbing',

while still believing in *displacement*:

'. . . the same basic process is operative when, regardless of how extreme or revolting an obsessive thought might be, it is still much less distressing than the idea it is covering up.'

As a personal view, we must add that nothing we have read convinces us that there is necessarily a hidden disturbing thought of this kind underlying obsessional thoughts.

Conditioning

Consider OCD from the viewpoint of conditioning and learning. In these terms, there might be a fundamental difference between what *instigated* the obsessions in the first place and what *maintains* them now. In terms of what instigated them, Hans Eysenck argued that neurotic behaviour is an example of faulty learning, an aberration of a perfectly useful process of learning, as described by the Russian physiologist Ivan Pavlov. The essence of Pavlovian conditioning is that a relationship is established between two otherwise unrelated events. In Pavlov's famous experiment, an association was formed between a bell and food, so that the sound of the bell was able to stimulate salivation. We can see that this is relevant to obsessions if we ask 'How does a normally ignored or innocuous situation (e.g. a milk-bottle top lying in the street, counting numbers) that evoked little fear or dread, now come to evoke disquiet, anxiety, dread or even terror?' Perhaps the best way of thinking about this is that there might be an element of accidental or chance association between one of a wide variety of thoughts and a mood. There are a number of cases reported in which the onset of obsessional disorder can apparently be traced to an association with a traumatic event.

Examples

A case of this kind was reported by John Woodard in 1757. Following a series of awful family traumas, a woman bearing her sixth child observed a porpoise in the river Thames. She was delighted with seeing this creature. Alas, some two weeks later, she suffered serious abdominal pain. At this point she recalled the porpoise and from then on was haunted by the obsessional fear that the animal would harm her baby.

Consider also the following case reported by G Skoog, which could fit the conditioning model.

A person has an attack of dizziness on his way home from work. After reaching home he opens the paper and sees the death announcements, and he faints. Some days later he feels tired and becomes dizzy. These feelings link themselves to the previous experiences, to situations of insecurity and to the possibility of death, with the development of a phobic obsessive syndrome as a result.

Gaining understanding

The nervous system is programmed to scan for causes of significant events and often gets the cause wrong. Hit your finger with a hammer, and you might blame your boss, or wife or children, even though they might have had nothing to do with it. Similarly, if you become ill after eating Thai food, you might well go off Thai food even though it had nothing to do with causing your illness. So, perhaps OCD is the outcome of a hypersensitive nervous system possessed by some human beings – a species known for its capacity to form odd associations between unrelated events.

The conditioning model certainly seems relevant to obsessions, but just how relevant it is, only time will tell. It is interesting to note that a wide range of situations can and do become candidates for obsessions. However, there are a number of particularly common themes, such as physical damage and contamination. The nervous system might be said to be 'prepared' to form certain associations and not others. For example, in the case of phobias, it could be argued that we are strongly prepared to develop spider and snake phobias and not prepared to learn, say, CD phobias.

Let's now consider the situation in which the obsession is well established. There might be an *incubation* of fear. Once acquired, fears can grow stronger with the passage of time. Each experience of the fear serves to strengthen it. Once the association is triggered by some chance event, it is self-reinforcing. A similar logic might be applicable to the origin of phobias.

Reinforcement and reward

Concerning what maintains obsessions, note that behaviour can also be changed, 'shaped', by techniques of reinforcement, described by B F Skinner. Reward appropriate behaviour, and we can train a rat to press a lever to obtain food or even teach a pigeon to steer a missile. Conversely, if negative consequences follow behaviour, the tendency is for the behaviour to stop, though this process is more complex.

Viewed in such terms, the origins of obsessional thoughts and much of compulsive behaviour might seem to make little sense. There is no obvious reward to the obsessional. Indeed, the obsessional might report extreme discomfort as a result of them and go to great lengths to get rid of them.

However, there are two crucially important qualifications to be added here. First, although the obsessions themselves might bring only pain, some temporary relief from this pain might be gained by the associated compulsive activity. As noted earlier, compulsive activity (the 'counter-reaction') can take the form of either behaviour (e.g. washing) or a mental activity (thinking thoughts that help to counter the obsession). Although such activity might be harmful in the long run, the *immediate* association might be with some very temporary gain. In this sense, the compulsive activity could be said to be 'reinforcing the obsession', i.e. making it more likely to occur in the future. Hence, the logic is suggested that the person should try to stop engaging in any such counter-reactions. Suppose that the obsession is about having acquired AIDS from touching a dirty surface. The counter-reaction might take the form of, for example, the overt behaviours of scrubbing the skin or searching libraries for medical books to bring reassurance. In addition, or instead, there might be mental compulsions such as trying to argue with the obsession or pleading with God. To break the reinforcement cycle, the person might then need to try to stop all such actions and gain exposure to the obsessional doubt.

As a further consideration, in terms of family life, we need to consider that some forms of compulsive behaviour can involve subtle social reinforcement. The behaviour can serve to manipulate family members. In some cases, family members can unwittingly help to maintain the behaviour by, for example, complying with the wilder excesses of the obsessive-compulsive's demands or giving repeated reassurance.

Mood state

Obsessions about unambiguously negative themes, such as death and injury, can fit an explanatory model in which a negative mood accentuates certain negative thoughts. Thus we might see the phenomenon in terms of an exaggeration of a normal brain process that links moods to thoughts. There might be a kind of mutual support between the thought, or *cognition*, and mood. For example, stress (discussed below) of a general kind, not necessarily caused by events related to the specific content of the obsession, might accentuate the specific thought, and so the vicious circle would continue.

Some studies have shown that obsessionals are more likely to be affected badly by depression and hostility, rather than by anxiety. Occasionally, women experience obsessions only at the time of menstruation. (Someone under unwanted stress is more likely to become depressed.) As the vicious circle is repeated, a broader range of stimuli in the environment might become associated with the circle, so as to be able to trigger it. It might be relevant in this context to note that obsessionals often find that a change of environment can bring temporary relief.

Viewing obsessions in this way suggests that probing the initial cause of the vicious circle is unlikely to be fruitful exercise. Rather, it is possible that all that can meaningfully be looked at is how the circle can be broken.

Stress

M Horowitz reported an experiment in which groups of 'normal' people watched films judged to be stress-inducing. The background to this experiment was the observation that, following a traumatic experience, many people report intrusive thoughts and nightmares. In the experiment, intrusive, distracting thoughts increased after watching a gory, stress-evoking film, as compared with a neutral film. A film with a depressing theme also aroused unwanted intrusions. That links in with normal life, where, in times of sadness, intrusive thoughts are more frequent.

A situation of natural stress also was studied. Mothers whose children were admitted into hospital for surgery were observed. Unpleasant and intrusive thoughts were more frequent in them than in a 'control' group of mothers. Similarly, war veterans have reported an increased frequency after exposure to the stress of combat.

The phenomena of nightmares and night terrors might also provide a useful lead here. Stress increases the severity and frequency of nightmares. In my (F.T.'s) experience, night terrors were more frequent at times of stress, such as when I was trying to make an important decision. Although the stress was not caused by any death-related events, it seemed to be accentuating the death-related night terrors.

Is my brain malfunctioning or damaged?

Obsessional disorder is usually described as a 'psychiatric condition' or 'psychological disorder'. What exactly do such terms mean? In what sense do they convey a meaning that distinguishes this disorder from, say, a liver disease or the result of physical damage to the brain as in a gunshot injury? In one form or another, such questions have occupied the minds of philosophers and scientists for a very long time. Alas, we can only give a very brief and necessarily superficial account of this issue here.

Some might say that obsessional disorder is a malfunction of the mind whereas the injury from a gunshot reflects a disorder of the physical brain. However, any such neat dichotomy between mind and brain raises more questions than answers. By 'psychiatric' and 'psychological' we refer here to phenomena concerned with how the brain processes information. Some of this processing is available to us in the form of the content of our conscious mind but much of it goes on at a subconscious level. The line that we adopt in this book fits a contemporary understanding within the brain and psychological sciences: obsessional disorder reflects a malfunction of both mind and brain, in that we cannot view the one without the other. In other words, the disorder has two aspects, mental (relating to the mind) and physical (relating to the brain). We might like to view psychotherapy as targeting the mental aspect and drugs as targeting the physical aspect but in reality the two are inseparable.

The computer model (or 'analogy')

Consider the computer analogy and the situation where something goes wrong in the way that a computer works. A vital caution to note about analogies is that they are no more than analogies. They are examples that are in some way similar in their working to the system under investigation; they are *not* identical, so sooner or later we will doubtless find their explanatory value limited. For example, some would argue that the computer analogy doesn't begin to do justice to the richness of the human brain, mind and experience. Nevertheless, such a 'simple' analogy might help us initially to ask relevant questions and clarify our thinking.

Broadly, we could identify two classes of reason as to why a computer might malfunction:

- There could be something wrong with the computer itself: some of its circuits might have been put together wrongly or someone with a pair of wire-cutters might have tampered with it. A sharp-eyed computer engineer might be able to spot the defect simply by examining the computer itself, without even plugging it in and switching on the power. The defect means that the computer gives a bizarre output even though appropriate information is fed into it, and it might be necessary to return the machine to the manufacturer.

- Alternatively, it might be a perfectly intact computer; there is nothing defective to be seen. Rather, something could be wrong with the program that is being run on the machine; in computer jargon, 'there is a bug in the program'. Or the user might be pressing the wrong buttons. A secretary rather than an engineer could solve the problem.

To pursue this analogy, current thinking is that in obsessional disorder there is a physical abnormality in the brain, which is manifest in abnormal processing of information. This is experienced as abnormal thought processes and behaviour.

Brain abnormality

Consider the notion that there might be some physical abnormality, such as brain damage or a hormone excess or deficiency, underlying obsessional disorder. There are reports in scientific publications of the onset of obsessional disorder immediately after traumatic injury to the head or accompanying the onset of epilepsy. Some investigators even believe that traumatic birth contributes to the condition. A survey on some patients in Chichester did indeed find an increased incidence of reported traumatic birth in the obsessional group, as compared to a control group. However, even if this relationship were firmly established, we would not be able to conclude unambiguously that obsessionals had suffered brain damage. An alternative explanation might be that, in traumatic cases, mother and baby were separated immediately after birth, but this could have implications for the structure of the growing brain. For a more zany explanation, some writers appeal to memory: the obsessional remembers the 'agony of being born'.

There is some evidence of brain abnormality in obsessionals, specifically (for the technically minded) in the temporal and parietal regions and the striatum. There seem to be some abnormalities in the patterns of electrical activity of the brain, the electroencephalogram (EEG). Map reading and spatial skills (e.g. the capacity to navigate) are said to be deficient (they certainly are in F.T.'s case!). Some surveys have found that obsessionals are more likely to be left-handed. Tantalisingly, there is also some evidence for temporal lobe disorder in people who have night terrors. Whether or not it confirms brain damage, the connection between sleep disorder and obsessional illness might prove revealing: the sleep of obsessive compulsive people is certainly abnormal.

Probing the brain

Using sophisticated technical equipment, it is possible to form an image of the activity of the various parts of the brain without any surgical intervention. Such studies reveal abnormalities in the brains of people with OCD. Certain regions are consistently found to be overactive, when compared with people who do not have the condition. Also when treatment (e.g. 'brain lock') is successful, the activity in these regions returns to a normal value. This profile of overactivity indicates a biological basis to the exaggerated thought processes of sufferers.

Patients can gain comfort from knowing about the biological basis of their disorder. Indeed, in the 'brain lock' treatment pioneered at the University of California, Los Angeles, by Dr Jeffrey Schwartz and colleagues (see Chapter 15), patients are shown recordings of their brains and the areas of overactivity pointed out. They then find it useful to try to visualise a particular set of brain cells 'working overtime' (firing in bursts of unusually high activity) and accept that this provides a rational basis to their distress. They are not evil or weak-willed people or guilty for their lot in life but are suffering from a 'respectable' medical disorder. Even if the images are unacceptable (e.g. violent and/or perverse sexual themes), they can be understood as the product of faulty brain mechanisms. The fault is one shared with very many other people.

To return to our analogy with a computer, does such evidence point to a fault of the kind an engineer might be asked to solve or one for which a secretary is most relevant? Maybe the truth lies somewhere with each feature of the analogy, which points to the added complexity of the brain as compared with a computer. There does seem to be something analogous to faulty wiring. However, the effects of this might sometimes be cured by changing behaviour or thoughts, analogous to rewriting the program.

The serotonin hypothesis

Another possible means to gaining insight into the abnormality concerns the chemical state of the brain, the activities of its transmitter substances that convey signals from one neuron (nerve cell) to another. Based on the therapeutic success of drugs (e.g. clomipramine) with obsessionals, there seems to be an abnormality in one of the brain's chemical messengers. Such drugs seem to restore the normal level of this messenger at certain key sites. Other drugs, effective against depression but that do not affect this messenger, do not help to combat OCD.

This hypothesis is thus based on the observation that the drugs that are successful in treating obsessional disorder specifically alter the levels of this one particular natural chemical messenger (also termed 'transmitter') used by the brain to communicate signals from one neuron to another. This transmitter is called serotonin (also 5-hydroxytriptamine or '5-HT'). This known effect of drugs has led to what is termed the *serotonin hypothesis* of OCD. (Effective drugs are called 'selective serotonin reuptake inhibitors', or SSRIs.) That is to say, the disorder's biological basis is one of faulty regulation of the level of this particular transmitter substance. The hypothesis is not a rival for the truth when considered against the evidence of overactivity in certain brain regions. Rather, the overactivity could well be another aspect of the same abnormality. The overactive regions could be the same ones that have abnormal levels of serotonin.

Researchers are justified in feeling some pride in establishing the serotonin hypothesis. Indeed, it reflects one of the more robust findings in psychiatric research. However, they are not sitting back relaxed with this finding. Not everyone responds to drugs that target serotonin, so other factors also seem to be implicated. Further research is being pursued.

Conscious and unconscious processing

In OCD, any biological disorder manifests itself as a psychological symptom. In the latter terms, one approach to understanding obsessional disorder is to consider the normal division of responsibility between conscious and subconscious processing of information by the brain. This perspective on obsessional disorder was introduced by Dan Stein, Naomi Fineberg and Soraya Seedat by comparing it with learning to ride a bicycle. If you have not yet mastered this task, you can surely relate the argument to any of a host of other tasks that have exactly the same principle, such as driving a car.

Can you recall the first time that you tried to ride a bicycle? Doubtless, as you first set off you were highly concentrated on the task, focused on just this one thing to the exclusion of everything else. As you and the bicycle started to wobble in an unsteady way, all of the 'mental energy' that you could muster was in the service of staying upright. Compare this novice performance with skilled cycling. You can now cycle and talk to a friend at the same time or observe the passing fields, listen to music on head-phones and take a drink. What has happened over the time since those first tentative steps? You still need to co-ordinate your eyes, balance organs and the muscles of your body in staying upright. However, these tasks are now performed at a subconscious level. Your conscious processing is occupied with other information processing, such as interpreting the significance of what your cycling companion is telling you. What once engaged conscious processing later moves to a subconscious level.

Suppose now that there is ice on the road and you start to slip and slide. The chances are that you will feel a powerful emotion – let's call it fear – and you will immediately stop talking to your companion. You will focus on the task of staying upright. The emotion of fear has changed the level of processing and all your conscious resources are now engaged with the single highest priority task.

This example illustrates several things relevant to our discussion:

- that information processing can occur at different levels, in this case described as conscious and subconscious;

- that the level at which processing occurs can change;

- that a strong emotion such as fear can change the priorities and level of processing.

The relevance of this to obsessions could be something like as follows. Normally, as we negotiate our way around the world we are bombarded by information about the outside world: smells, sounds and sights. Most of this information processing probably never reaches our conscious awareness. It is just as well that it doesn't, because our consciousness would be inundated with information. Chaos would be the result. To most people, even passing a cemetery does not trigger a sequence of conscious processing, though it is registered at some level by the brain.

In OCD, certain bits of information get tagged as important and occupy conscious processing. Anxiety is the result, which sets up a vicious circle. Anxiety labels them as even more important, which brings them more often into conscious awareness, which increases the strength of negative emotion attached to them, and so on. But why does one particular thought get treated in this way? We don't know but some possibilities can be suggested:

- It could just be chance, as described earlier in this chapter. The thought happens to occur at a time of stress and gets labelled as important and deserving of further attention, and so the brain's cycle gets going.

- In other cases, the thought might relate to a particular concern that was already quite strongly labelled as negative, such as death-related themes or a range of unacceptable sexual acts.

Another way of looking at this is that the subconscious processing is unable to find a resolution to the problem and so the content of the obsession regularly pops into consciousness for further mental work to be done on it. Appropriate external triggers such as passing a cemetery also start the sequence going. This also makes sense from general experience. Suppose that a non-obsessional or obsessional person quite naturally has a problem to solve, such as how to avoid going into the red in the bank. This tends to occupy the person's awareness, no matter how much they try to avoid it. It just keeps popping into awareness or is triggered by money-related events, and this is also what the obsessional thought appears to do.

A feedback explanation of obsessional disorder?

In 1985, a new explanation of obsessional disorder appeared, based on 'negative feedback', long familiar to engineers. It fits the other perspectives just described.

Another analogy

The everyday examples of negative feedback control are legion. Take the thermostat that helps regulate the temperature of a room. The room's occupant returns from holiday, and the room temperature is, say, 15°C. He sets the thermostat at 20°C and switches the heating on. The setting of 20°C constitutes the *set-point* or *goal* of the system. The temperature of 15°C is the *actual* value of room temperature. In effect, the thermostat compares the goal with the actual value, and the system sets in motion action to bring the actual value to the goal value. When the room temperature reaches 20°C, actual temperature and the goal temperature are equal and the heating action switches off. If the room temperature falls, heating is automatically switched on to bring it back to 20°C. The system is called 'feedback' because the actual state is fed back and compared with the desired state. It is called *negative* feedback because any difference, or deviation, between goal and actual state tends to be *self-eliminating*. Deviation drives the system so as to eliminate deviation.

Application to the disorder

Let us take the situation of hand-washing. There is a goal, a criterion of cleanliness that is being strived for. The actual state of cleanliness, as perceived by the individual, is compared with this desired state. For most of us, we rapidly reach our goal. The difference between desired state and perceived actual state is soon eliminated, and we turn the tap off and then grab a towel. According to the feedback model, it is useful to see the compulsive hand-washer as someone who is striving unsuccessfully to reach the goal of cleanliness. The feedback pathway and comparison process are abnormal. Desired state is compared with the *perception* of actual state, but for the compulsive hand-washer the hands are perceived as still contaminated. The notion of contamination occupies conscious awareness for an excessive amount of time. In such terms, the fundamental problem in OCD is a mismatch between what is desired and what is achieved.

In the context of negative feedback systems, a comment on the relentless pursuit of thinness by people with anorexia might well also prove relevant. They never achieve their goal because they are never able to recognise that they are, in fact, thin. This goal engages consciousness for inordinate lengths of time.

Insight

This model of OCD immediately offers possible insight. For example, rather than simply asking what makes people compulsively wash their hands, sometimes it might be appropriate also to ask what prevents them from stopping and switching to the next logical activity. Indeed, in general there is nothing so abnormal about hand-washing; it is the length of time the obsessional devotes to it that is abnormal. Furthermore, from discussions with some compulsive hand-washers, it would seem that they experience distress not so much when they start washing but at not being able to stop. They do not feel that they are under the control of some omnipotent force, but are frustrated by their lack of will in not being able to quit. One might see here why therapists can sometimes help their patients by specifying a criterion of when to quit. For example, 'Rather than wash for four hours, wash for only three hours at first.' The therapist is providing the needed feedback, the criterion of completion.

The condition called *primary obsessional slowness* might also be understood in these terms. For example, an obsessional might simply take an inordinately long time to get dressed but would not be trying to avoid some harmful or catastrophic outcome. In such terms the person would find it very difficult to reach the goal 'I am now correctly dressed'.

Occasionally it has been maintained that there is a link between obsessional disorder and the conditions of stuttering and stammering. Although it is sometimes suggested that stutterers have a tendency to be obsessional, we know of no reliable evidence on this point. It is very tempting to speculate here, given that the essence of stuttering is a failure in a negative feedback system: the stutterer has inadequate feedback from the spoken sound to continue normal speech production and 'gets stuck'.

A negative feedback model would seem to give more insight than some other possible models. It emphasises that compulsive behaviour is not something that is generated purely internally by a build-up of energy or simply by a defective bit of the brain's machinery (albeit malfunction here is suggested, as discussed earlier). Rather, the experience of compulsion and the associated behaviour arise in the obsessionals' interaction with their environment. The system is not like a pressure cooker that has to let off steam once in a while to maintain internal pressure within safe limits. Stopping the compulsive behaviour would not be expected to lead to a build-up of pressure that will cause trouble elsewhere. It would not be like jamming up the outlet of a pressure cooker, which would be expected to result in the appliance 'exploding'.

Under the directions of a therapist, the obsessional is able to refrain from engaging in compulsive behaviour with no harmful effects. On a longer time-scale, curing a compulsive disorder would not be expected to lead to problems elsewhere – to the condition called *symptom substitution*. It is not as if some kind of psychic energy must be discharged somewhere and the compulsive behaviour is the vehicle for this, as suggested by Freud. The fact that symptom substitution does not occur following the behavioural treatment of compulsive disorder is an argument against the Freudian model of neurosis.

Conflict

The negative feedback model provides insight into the indecisiveness of the obsessional. This is characterised as two control systems being in conflict. Bearing this analogy in mind, consider 21-year-old Hank, reported by R K Pitman.

Hank needed to spend 15 minutes adjusting water temperature before taking a shower. Fine adjustments were made to get things 'just right'. On one occasion, a friend asked Hank to go to a baseball game. Hank in fact wanted to visit a racetrack, but agreed to go with the friend to the baseball game. Hank drove his friend towards the baseball game, but as they got nearer, Hank's urge to be at the racetrack grew. Much to the friend's disappointment, Hank turned the car around and drove towards the racetrack. However, as the racetrack got nearer, so Hank's guilt intensified. He again turned the car around and pursued the original course. A series of such oscillations was ended by Hank parking the car midway between the two goals, at which point the friend took over the driving.

Hank also reported great difficulty in ordering from a menu when there was more than one desirable dish. The waiter would end up moving between Hank and the kitchen in response to Hank's vacillations of desire. Each time a choice was made, attention was soon shifted from the chosen item to the unchosen one, which then competed for dominance.

Goal-seeking

There is another interesting general feature of the negative feedback model. Consider a man at a fete trying his skill in not letting the two bits of wire touch each other. Watch his exact movements as he has two or three goes at it. The goal is always the same, to steer the loop along a middle course. However, on close examination, it will be seen that the actual movements are different from game to game. The behaviour is not stereotyped. He will try slightly different strategies as he gets better at it. This is like the obsessional: typically, he will use different hand movements, different ways of rubbing the soap, but always striving for a match with the same goal of perfect cleanliness. Similarly, the compulsive counter will try different mental tricks to reach perfection.

The obsessive-compulsive is often acting logically in terms of attempting to gain control. Hand-washing is a logical action suggested by the perception of contaminated hands. In 'normal' people, and indeed for the obsessional before the onset of the disorder, the action of washing would generate negative feedback to alter the perception of dirtiness or contamination to one of cleanliness. However, under obsessional conditions the perception does not change with effort exerted; normal feedback does not occur and the system is said to have gone *open-loop*. Worse still, the system can generate a vicious circle, known also as exhibiting *positive feedback*. That is to say, the longer obsessionals wash their hands, the more they perceive them to be contaminated, and so the more they wash them, and . . . . Anxiety might even increase in parallel. How do they ever manage to stop? We can imagine that, after hours of washing, another goal will be able to take control, such as the growing attraction of sleep as a result of exhaustion or the fear of future exhaustion.

Obsessions without compulsive behaviour

F.T.'s experience

For my own (F.T.'s) obsessional thoughts, let us speculate: the two bits of information – desired and actual – are compared in an attempt to eliminate a disparity. The evidence is based largely on my own experience. As we have said elsewhere in this book, the intrusions often came in response to situations that in some sense highlighted disparity. Stimuli confirming the transitory nature of existence were commonly triggers, but so were the diametrically opposite class of situations underlining the present and future goodness of life. Information relevant to future attainment was a strong trigger to death themes, such as:

cue – 'You speak good German' → *mental response* – successful assimilation into Germany during my future study leave.

By contrast, pieces of information relevant to the past (e.g. 'what a great summer school in 1986') were not trigger cues, unless they served to trigger an intermediate thought sequence:

'1986' → 'seems like yesterday' → 'time flies' → 'can't stop it' with an accompanying negative emotion.

My feeling was that, where two bits of information are incongruous, triggering the one can serve to excite the other. The system then searches for the possibilities for correcting the disparity. When my lifestyle and prospects were not so good, as on returning from Denmark, the intrusions were very much less intense.

Some famous insights

Although my (F.T.'s) observations arise from my own mind, I am not alone in thinking along these lines. Pierre Janet used the expression *l'association par contraste* to describe a very similar phenomenon, and noted that, for example, loving parents would often be obsessed with the thought of selling their loved ones to the devil or mutilating them with a knife. The latter was particularly common among his patients. Janet also discussed the blasphemous thoughts of John Bunyan, which were experienced in a religious context, as an example of obsessions acting in opposition to the current intention. My own self-observations in this area also coincide with those reported by the 19th-century writer Thomas de Quincey. In his classic, *Confessions of an English Opium-Eater*, de Quincey recorded:

'. . . the exuberant and riotous prodigality of life naturally forces the mind more powerfully upon the antagonist thought of death, and the wintry sterility of the grave. For it may be observed generally that, wherever two thoughts stand related to each other by a law of antagonism, and exist, as it were, by mutual repulsion, they are apt to suggest each other. On these accounts it is that I find it impossible to banish the thought of death when I am walking alone in the endless days of summer; and any particular death, if not actually more affecting, at least haunts my mind more obstinately and besiegingly, in that season.'

Such observations suggest that this type of sufferer might unfortunately also need to do some work on their positive thought sequences. They might thereby be able to pre-empt the appearance of the negative thoughts. For example, suppose that a beautiful summer's day has been regularly associated with the thought sequence 'the world is wonderful . . . but it will not last'. In this case, the thinker might try to change the thought 'the world is wonderful' into something like 'so, things seem just about OK'.

Obsessional thoughts and compulsive behaviour

How does compulsive behaviour become associated with obsessional thoughts? We suggest that there are several ways. First, the behaviour might be acquired somewhat arbitrarily as a trick for stopping a thought, or at least reducing its intensity. As an example of this, consider Linda, reported by D Hill:

> Linda was a highly intelligent 47-year-old teacher who, for 36 years, had experienced compulsive thoughts and rituals. At the age of 10 she was preoccupied with a passage from the Bible: 'to blaspheme against the Holy Ghost is unforgivable'. Later she was to be troubled by the intrusion of such words as 'damn' and 'bloody' into her consciousness. Linda discovered that the anxiety that these thoughts evoked could be reduced to some extent by repeating an apparently arbitrary activity a set number of times. When she was 13 years old, the intrusive words were of a sexual nature and she was obsessed by the thought of sexual relations with the Holy Ghost. Again though, repetitive acts, such as walking up and down the stairs, served to allay the anxiety.

We suggest that such arbitrary rituals are analogous to mental rituals in that they are acquired by trial and error and retained because they serve, in the short term, to allay the discomfort.

In other cases, rather than arbitrary activity the behaviour might be one that had usually been performed quite normally in solving problems similar to that presented by the obsessional thought. For example, washing of some sort is a usual response to the perception of dirt or impurity, both physical and, in some cases, moral. There are such sayings as 'cleanse yourself of sin' and 'wash your mouth out for saying that'. Checking by means of inspection, seeking personal reassurance or making a telephone call are perfectly normal responses to uncertainty. These actions only become abnormal because of the intensity and frequency with which they are performed. We believe that such extensive behaviour is like obsessional rumination. It is not arbitrary and, although grossly exaggerated and ultimately fruitless, it represents a natural and logical means of trying to find a solution.

Sometimes people will view their compulsive behaviour as providing information relevant to the obsessional rumination, presumably via some supernatural route. Pierre Janet saw a number of patients of this kind. For example, Vy was tormented by doubts as to whether he really believed in God. In walking the streets, he felt that relevant information could be generated by observing whether he was able to avoid treading on the shadows of trees. If he succeeded, this was a sign that he believed in God. If he failed, this indicated non-belief.

Creativity

How is it that obsessionals are often creative? The obsessional trait of dogged persistence is sometimes seen as blind obedience to a fixed course of action, the exact opposite of what is needed for creativity. Perhaps obsessionals set high, indeed perfectionist, goals that they attempt to reach by a variety of strategies. Did such writers as Swift ruminate endlessly, trying to match an actual phrase to an idealised state? Investigating the creative talent and working style of obsessionals could be useful. We have a good account of John Bunyan's thought processes, in his work *Grace Abounding to the Chief of Sinners*. We know that Bunyan was a formidable hair-splitter. Convinced that he had committed the ultimate sin, that against the Holy Ghost, he tried countless times to match his sin against those recorded in the Bible. Each time he failed, finding ever more original reasons why his own sin was worse. In other words, his neutralising thoughts were always inadequate. Each novel approach led to the same conclusion:

> 'This one consideration would always kill my Heart, *My sin was point-blank against my Saviour*, and that too, at that height, that I had in my heart said of him, *Let him go if he will*. Oh! me thoughts, this sin was bigger than the sins of a Countrey, of a Kingdom, or of the whole

World, no one pardonable, nor all of them together, was able to equal mine, mine out-went them every one.'

In this quotation we see good examples of the tendency to categorise in extremes rather than shades of grey and the perfectionism of some obsessionals. However, we imagine that a mental process by which ideas are compared against a perfectionist standard would, if anything, be compatible with creativity.

Anthony Storr reached a similar conclusion, believing that some types of creativity are related to the obsessional's wish for order. A fact that does not match current scientific thought can cause the same irritation as the crooked picture, the dirt in the corner or the clothes dropped on the floor. It is something outside the ordered scheme, and therefore out of control. Storr argued that the pursuit of science has something of an obsessional activity about it. Advance in science depends on producing theories that can account for otherwise unaccountable findings. He noted the case of a scientist who would make the angry comment 'I'll beat the bastard' in the face of technical problems.

The tendency to what is called *over-inclusion* has been noted in creativity. This refers to a tendency to attend to information that might seem to be irrelevant to the task in hand. The similarity of this to obsessional thinking hardly needs pointing out! The production of major creative work involves the use of imagery and metaphor, and in these capacities the obsessional is well represented. Highly creative musicians have a tendency toward solitary hobbies and individualistic creative activity.

In summary, obsessional disorder remains in some respects an enigma, and it would be foolish to try to dress it up to be otherwise. However, there are a few leads and we believe the discovery of abnormalities in the brain and the feedback model (see 'A feedback explanation of obsessional disorder?', earlier) to be the most promising.

17
Some famous thoughts

'O God, grant me repentence, grant me reformation. Grant that I may be no longer disturbed with doubts and harassed with vain terrours.'
SAMUEL JOHNSON, *Prayers and Meditations*,
29 March 1766

Here we look at some famous people whose lives can help our understanding of obsessions. It might also be that you can gain some help from looking at the lives of others with similar experiences or whose writings are relevant. One function that this chapter could serve for you is to destroy forever any notion that OCD is a sign of failure or weak will. In it you will find famous scientists, musicians and writers who either suffered seriously from the condition or at least showed strongly obsessional characteristics in their behaviour. (Dickens is described on the website.) Alas, we were unable to find more than one famous obsessional woman to write about (Karen Carpenter), though Dr Jeffrey Schwartz mentions the possibility of the actress, Katherine Hepburn. Howard Hughes apparently told her that, for a woman who took 18 showers a day, she was in no position to ridicule his obsessions!

Samuel Johnson (1709–1784)

Researchers into Johnson are fortunate in having what is perhaps the most famous biography of all time, James Boswell's *The Life of Samuel Johnson*, where they can find in detail what Johnson liked, disliked, ate, drank, thought and feared. Boswell's work, a brilliant insight into the mind and behaviour of one man, is itself a classic of English literature. We might well know more about Johnson than about any other person who ever lived.

The interaction between the two men is especially revealing: the prudish and 'very English' Johnson and the much younger and usually more liberal-minded upper-class Scotsman Boswell, who had earlier tasted the temptations of London and caught venereal disease. Boswell gives a vivid account of their regular meetings, dining at the Mitre Tavern, where he soaked up the wisdom of Johnson, such as 'Endeavour to be as perfect as you can in every respect'.

Although Johnson at times comes across as 'holier than thou' and dogmatic, he managed to blend the qualities of kindness, genius and clowning. He gave insight to every situation, profound and trivial. So often one feels 'If only I had thought to say that.' For example, on being asked by a woman to account for a mistake in the dictionary he had written, Johnson offered the incomparable 'Ignorance, Madam, pure ignorance'. We can think of occasions, while teaching, when we would have been well served to have had that particular expression available!

Childhood

Samuel Johnson ('Dr Johnson') – writer, poet, critic, sage, philosopher, biographer, moralist, wit, formidable debater and conversationalist *extraordinaire* – was born into a humble household in Lichfield in 1709. The birth was a very difficult one. His father was a not-very-successful bookseller and suffered from melancholy. Mrs Johnson could be characterised as having more than average anxiety. Samuel felt that he inherited his own tendency to melancholy, a 'vile temperament', from his father.

At an early age, the boy was instructed by his somewhat stern and over-scrupulous mother on the two possible fates that await the soul: heaven or torment. It is not difficult to see the family as a fertile breeding ground for Samuel's later agonies of guilt. At school, the young Samuel showed himself to have a desire to excel, an incredibly good memory (which he also had later in life) and to be competitive, but curiously to have also a streak of indolence.

He didn't join in activities with other pupils, though his incomparable intellect was held in awe by his fellows. One day, while sitting alone at home reading *Hamlet*, he was so overcome by fear of the ghost that he moved nearer to the door that opened to the street. Samuel would spend hours wandering the fields and lanes around Lichfield, preferably in the company of a companion, Hector. However, Samuel's lengthy speeches were not addressed to Hector as part of a normal interaction, but represented thinking aloud. Samuel showed some signs of rebellion about going to the same church as his parents. Boswell noted that, at the age of 10, Samuel's mind was disturbed by 'scruples of infidelity, which preyed upon his spirits, and made him very uneasy' and '. . . he began to think himself highly culpable for neglecting such a means of information, and took himself severely to task for this sin, adding many acts of voluntary, and to others unknown, penance'.

The young man

Johnson gained a place at Oxford University, but tragically because he didn't have enough money he was unable to remain a student. To his immense disappointment, he was forced to return to Lichfield. Without any logical reason, Johnson blamed himself. He came near to suicide and feared for his sanity. Intense anxiety was accompanied by feelings of hopelessness and helplessness. From accounts of Johnson's later cycles of behaviour, between the lows of inactivity and the highs of extreme exertion, he might be described as manic–depressive. Periods of idleness, characterised by daydreaming, would be interrupted by fanatical concentration and incredible energy. Boswell noted that 'A horrour at life in general is more consonant with Johnson's habitual gloomy cast of thought.'

The adult Dr Johnson

In case you should suppose that psychiatric problems are associated with only the tender and the meek, Johnson disconfirms this. In physique, he was by all accounts about as feeble and weak as a full-grown grizzly bear!

Johnson had tics and various other compulsive mannerisms; on occasion he was the object of some ridicule in public. Years later, on the subject of these movements, Boswell quoted a letter from Sir Joshua Reynolds:

> 'These motions or tricks of Dr Johnson are improperly called convulsions. He could sit motionless, when he was told to do so, as well as any other man; my opinion is that it proceeded from a habit which he had indulged himself in, of accompanying his thoughts with certain untoward actions, and those actions always appeared to me as if they were meant to reprobate some part of his past conduct. Whenever he was not engaged in conversation, such thoughts were sure to rush into his mind; and for this reason, any company, any employment, whatever, he preferred to being alone . . .'

In 1737, Johnson and a friend, David Garrick (later to achieve fame in the theatre), left Lichfield to make the 120-mile journey to London, into the unknown. Life in the capital was not easy for Johnson, at first leading a precarious existence as a hack-writer. However, the city's ceaseless stimulation afforded him some escape from ruminations about guilt. Estranged from his wife towards whom he felt great responsibility and guilt, Johnson led something of a waif's life for a while.

His behaviour was exemplary, showing great financial generosity not only to his wife but also to almost anyone in need. Johnson collected a circle of misfits and eccentrics, with whom he would spend long hours. His close friend Mrs Thrale described how Johnson 'nursed whole nests of people in his house, where the lame, the blind, the sick, and the sorrowful found a sure retreat from all the evils whence his little income could secure them'.

The obsessional trait of accuracy and meticulousness, an ability to 'split hairs', was put to good use by Johnson in producing his dictionary. He insisted on exact use of rules and words. For instance, he criticised Boswell for saying 'to make money', insisting that this implied to *coin* money. In Boswell's words, Johnson's students were urged to show 'perpetual vigilance against the slightest degrees of falsehood'.

Boswell described a scene concerning Johnson in his thirties, at a stage in his life when he had already written speeches for foremost politicians. Johnson had been asked to dine at the home of Edward Cave, and another distinguished guest, Walter Harte, had been invited. On arriving, Johnson felt ashamed of his shabby clothes, so before the other guest arrived, hid himself behind a screen, where later his meal was surreptitiously served. During the meal, Harte praised a recent book that Johnson had written. Cave was later to explain to Harte how happy his comments had made the invisible Johnson dining behind the screen.

Johnson found a poor woman lying exhausted in the street and unable to walk. He promptly lifted the unfortunate soul onto his back and carried her to his house, whereupon he discovered that she was a prostitute. Johnson cared for her until she was well and then tried to point her towards what he considered to be a virtuous occupation. He was known to enjoy the company of such women, though feeling great pity for their lot in life. This observation, and the fact that he kept some very disreputable male company, has raised the question as to whether he ever gave in to temptation. Our guess is not, but of course we cannot be sure. We know that he had to stop visiting David Garrick at Drury Lane theatre, the reason being simple: given Johnson's uncompromising moral principles, he couldn't bear the sexual passion aroused by Garrick's actress companions.

Johnson's reputation as a skilled raconteur is beautifully illustrated in Boswell's biography:

'. . . he had accumulated a great fund of miscellaneous knowledge, which, by a peculiar promptitude of mind, was ever ready at his call, and which he constantly accustomed himself to clothe in the most apt and energetick expression. Sir Joshua Reynolds once asked him by what means he had attained his extraordinary accuracy and flow of language. He told him that he had early laid it down as a fixed rule to do his best on every occasion, and in every company; to impart whatever he knew in the most forcible language he could put it in; and that by constant practice, and never suffering any careless expressions to escape him, or attempting to deliver his thoughts without arranging them in the clearest manner, it became habitual to him.'

Sir Aubrey Lewis noted that he was impressed by how often some of his obsessional patients complained of the need to repeat to themselves all that they heard and to formulate precisely how to express their own thoughts.

Profound insight into obsessionality

As an account of intrusive thoughts, it would be difficult to improve upon Johnson's:

'. . . an irresistible obtrusion of a disagreeable image, which you always wished away, but could not dismiss, an incessant persecution of a troublesome thought, neither to be pacified nor ejected. Such has of late been the state of my own mind. I had formerly great command of my attention, and what I did not like could forbear to think on . . .'

In addition to Boswell's biography, we have Johnson's *Prayers and Meditations*. These are very revealing of the obsessional personality, showing a mind gripped with guilt, doubts about worthiness, and fear of insanity and death. The same theme occurs again and again: the request for forgiveness from sin, strength to overcome indolence and, finally, a smooth transition to the after-life. So keen was Johnson to obtain eternal life that he even asked a man condemned to die at the gallows, a Dr Dodd, to make a last plea on his behalf when he reached 'the other side'.

Johnson managed beautifully to weave personally held fears and aspirations into his stories, a classic being *Rasselas*, the tale of an

Abyssinian prince who abandons the comforts of his palace to discover the secret of happiness. Rasselas searches far and wide, consulting a wide variety of people and seeing the wondrous sights of the world. He attends the lectures of distinguished philosophers at university, but alas finds that, in spite of eloquent academic arguments on the nature of happiness, in private their lives are as prone to grief as those of lesser mortals. Despairing of ever finding an answer, Rasselas asks the advice of a friendly and hospitable hermit living in a cave, only to discover that, lacking the opportunity for distraction, the unfortunate hermit is bombarded mercilessly with intrusive thoughts. The reader is expected to reach the conclusion that the elusive state of happiness is to be found not in this world but, God willing, in the next.

A striking contradiction in Johnson is the disparity between what he achieved and his own perception of his worth, on which so many of his obsessional thoughts concerning indolence turned. It is true that Johnson had phases of relative inactivity, but to all but a mind torn by the guilt of perfectionism these would fit very easily into context. His productivity defies belief: in just a few years, he produced a comprehensive dictionary, involving consideration of around 250,000 quotations. Yet Johnson still ruminated richly about his indolence.

Johnson displayed honesty and an intolerance for cant and affectation. For example, when a devout man, James Beattie, told Johnson that he had been '. . . at times troubled with impious thoughts', he got the reply 'If I was to divide my life into three parts, two of them have been filled with such thoughts'. Herein lies a paradox: that the obsessional, a person characterised by extreme persistence and dogged determination, could be so easily distracted from his goal by unwanted thoughts.

Johnson always hoped that things might get better. Boswell reported his saying that the present was never a happy time for any human being but that, because the future might reveal improved times, some happiness was produced by hope.

Johnson, who described himself as unsettled, as a 'kind of ship with a wide sail, and without an anchor', went on to argue that present happiness is possible only under the influence of alcohol. With the help of wine, he was able (in his own words) 'to get rid of myself, to send myself away'.

Johnson was determined not to be caught unawares by the future but he prepared himself for future disasters so effectively that this caused difficulty in enjoying the present. Walter Bate wrote that

Johnson tried to control the habit of 'anticipating evils', realising its insidious effect when carried too far. He tried to replace it with the 'habit of being pleased' but the former had become too much a part of his sense of identity.

Compulsive behaviour

Bate described Johnson's need to 'divide up' the jumble of his feelings and reduce them to manageable units, which we also see in his constant resort to arithmetic and counting. For example, he would blow out his breath loudly when he had finished a lengthy remark or argument, as though he were punctuating and ending it.

Johnson found that the exercise of mathematics provided great pleasure and some escape from painful ruminations on guilt and on the prospect of insanity and death.

Boswell described another compulsive behaviour of Johnson's:

'He had another peculiarity, of which none of his friends ever ventured to ask an explanation. It appeared to me some superstitious habit, which he contracted early, and from which he had never called upon his reason to disentangle him. This was his anxious care to go out or in at a door or passage by a certain number of steps from a certain point, or at least so as that either his right or his left foot (I am not certain which) should constantly make the first actual movement when he came close to the door or passage. Thus I conjecture: for I have, upon innumerable occasions, observed him suddenly stop, and then seem to count his steps with a deep earnestness; and when he had neglected or gone wrong in this sort of magical movement, I have seen him go back again, put himself in a proper posture to begin the ceremony, and, having gone through it, break from his abstraction, walk briskly on, and join his companion.'

With the help of an opera-glass, looking from a room in Bedford Street, a certain Mr S Whyte was able to observe Johnson in Henrietta Street:

'I perceived him at a good distance walking along with a peculiar solemnity of deportment, and an awkward sort of measured step. Upon every post as he passed along, he deliberately laid his hand; but missing one of them, when he had got at some distance, he seemed suddenly to recollect himself; and immediately returning carefully performed the accustomed ceremony, and resumed his former course, not omitting one till he gained the crossing.'

The passage of time

Johnson left a vivid record of his fear of the passage of time. For example:

'I have now begun the sixtieth year of my life. How the last year has past I am unwilling to terrify myself with thinking. This day has been passed in great perturbation. I was distracted at Church in an uncommon degree, and my distress has had very little intermission.'

On this same day he recorded in his *Prayers and Meditations*:

'This day it came into my mind to write the history of my melancholy. On this I purpose to deliberate; I know not whether it may not too much disturb me.'

In spite of the suffering experienced by Johnson, Boswell observed that he rarely, if ever, complained. In Boswell's own inimitable style 'What philosophick heroism was it in him to appear with such manly fortitude in the world, while he was inwardly so distressed!' He was much engaged by attempting the resolution of problems, whether personal or national, rather than whining about them.

We might see a dread of mortality in Johnson's comment to Sir Joshua Reynolds:

'It has often grieved me, Sir, to see so much mind as the science of painting requires, laid out upon such perishable materials: why do you not oftener make use of copper? I could wish your superiority in the art you profess to be preserved in stuff more durable than canvas.'

Time was particularly precious to Johnson in the context of getting older, something about which he hated to be reminded. Once, when he was confined to bed, he counted the days, which came to a total of 129: '. . . more than the third part of a year, and no inconsiderable part of human life'.

Johnson was disturbed when Boswell reminded a family with whom they were staying that it was Johnson's birthday – 18 September. The day '. . . fills me with thoughts which it seems to be the general care of humanity to escape'. The night before his 66th birthday, this time spent in France, was a sleepless one as Johnson wrestled with the implications of advancing years. His thoughts turned even more strongly to the meaning of life, the existence of evil and its relevance to the possibility of an after-life:

'It is scarcely to be imagined that Infinite Benevolance would create a being capable of enjoying so much more than is here to be enjoyed, and qualified by nature to prolong pain by remembrance and anticipate it by terror, if he was not designed for something nobler and better than a state, in which many of his faculties can serve only for his torment . . .'

Johnson showed exceptional courage in the face of danger, until seized by the prospect of death. Even when sailing in a tempest off Scotland, Johnson was observed to be lying in his bunk, quite calm and with a greyhound cushioned against his back to help him keep warm. The idea of death aroused his fear in a more abstract sense. He seemed to fear annihilation even more than the torments of hell. Although Johnson was a believer in the after-life, it was the *uncertainty* regarding his salvation that seemed to cause him most torment.

A friend from Lichfield, Anna Seward, tried to reason with him that annihilation was not something to fear: 'the dread of annihilation, which is only a pleasing dream'. He was, of course, unconvinced:

'It is neither pleasing nor sleep; it is nothing. Now mere existence is so much better than nothing that one would rather exist even in pain than not exist.'

Johnson's fear of annihilation led him to a great interest in supernatural phenomena, such as London's numerous ghost 'sightings', as possible evidence of life after death. We are reminded of Woody Allen's appeals in his films that God should give just one little sign of his presence.

In 1776, Boswell persuaded Johnson to discuss thought control or, as they termed it, 'management of the mind'. His answers are interesting from the viewpoint of modern psychotherapy: one must divert distressing thoughts, not fight them.' Boswell asked Johnson whether it was possible to 'think them down', and was told 'To attempt to think them down is madness'. We must agree with Johnson.

In 1779, Johnson was deeply moved by the death of David Garrick. He had memories of the day, 42 years earlier, when they had travelled to London, and was observed 'bathed in tears' at the funeral. Johnson had earlier denied that Garrick was ill; the mere possibility that a friend might die was unthinkable. He hated to part from any situation, as this had broader connotations, so when some good friends moved from Streatham to Brighton this seemed like a permanent 'goodbye'.

Just before his death, Johnson asked Sir John Hawkins where he would be buried. 'Doubtless in Westminster Abbey' was the reply. Johnson clearly had a feeling that this would be so. He had shown a reluctance to enter the Abbey over the preceding years but even in such a situation his wit did not desert him. On being asked by Lady Knight to join her for a visit to the Abbey, Johnson replied 'No, not while I can keep out'.

In the last hundred or so years, there have been several analyses of Johnson's condition. One, by P P Chase, contains an interesting speculation that Johnson's behavioural problems arose from the effects of lack of oxygen at birth. At times, in order to obtain peace of mind and body, Johnson took opium in sufficient quantities to become comatose. Boswell also reported that: 'Such was the heat and irritability of his blood that not only did he pare his nails to the quick but scraped the joints of his fingers with a pen-knife, till they seemed quite red and raw.' Never, though, in spite of all Johnson's physical and mental suffering, was death viewed as a welcome escape from pain. Johnson held on to life tenaciously.

George Henry Borrow (1803–1881)

George Borrow – author, explorer, linguist, animal lover and eccentric – gave some of the best accounts of obsessional disorder to be found anywhere. Borrow was born in 1803 in East Dereham, Norfolk, of a military family. He described his birth as being premature and troubled. In his autobiographical classic *Lavengro* (meaning 'wordmaster'), Borrow described himself as being 'born with excessive sensibility' and his life as characterised by 'wild imaginings and strange sensations'. An outsider from conventional society, Borrow didn't fit into the school system, preferring to learn things in his own way. He suffered from fits and, as a child, was gloomy, introspective and withdrawn, liable to burst into tears. His strange behaviour and failure to conform to accepted standards were a source of great worry and incredulity to his parents. In his own words, he liked:

'. . . to look upon the heavens, and to bask in the rays of the sun, or to sit beneath hedgerows and listen to the chirping of the birds, indulging the while in musing and meditation.'

He was later described consistently as being of striking good looks and physical appearance, very tall, and of extraordinary courage and physical endurance. His memory was most impressive, and he was sentimental and extremely superstitious. He loved ghost stories.

Both as a child and as an adult, Borrow was an enigma, strongly egotistic, a natural 'show-off' and yet hypochondriacal, someone spending enormous lengths of time on his own. In later years he suffered from serious depression, and contemplated suicide. He was a man of firm opinions, either liking someone intensely or disliking them intensely. His irritability, pride and stubbornness offended many people and even frightened some.

Borrow's biographer, Michael Collie, describes him as 'paranoid, secretive, uncommunicative and distrustful'. Even as a famous author, he was never at home in accepted and 'respectable' middle-class society, preferring instead the company of tramps, snake catchers, boxers, gypsies, criminals, down-and-outs and the assorted 'marginal' individuals that he frequently encountered while trekking around the world.

He had an incredible talent for foreign languages, and was reckoned to be one of the foremost linguists of his time. He acquired some languages by talking with gypsies, Irish peasants and other native speakers. His interest in Danish resulted from a fascination with wild and giant red-headed Vikings, aroused by seeing some Viking skulls. Borrow's learning technique stretched masochism to new lengths. He acquired a Bible written in Danish, and literally night after night was spent systematically comparing the words with those of an English Bible until he was fluent. By 18, he was said to have a good understanding of 12 languages, though the inevitable weaknesses of the self-taught were obvious when he translated English into a foreign tongue. Borrow was acquainted with 42 languages.

Working life

Borrow started his working life training to be a solicitor in Norwich, but abandoned this for the more exciting pastures of writing in London, printing Bibles in Russia and selling them in Spain. His invitation for an interview at the London office of the Bible Society illustrates Borrow's boundless energy. Arriving first thing in the morning, he waited on the doorstep, having walked the 112 miles from Norwich to London in 27½ hours and having spent fivepence-halfpenny on the way for one roll, two apples, a pint of ale and a glass of milk. Even more amazing is Borrow's well-documented experience in Russia. For an Englishman with no formal linguistic qualifications to teach himself Manchu in a few months would sound impressive. To then translate the Bible into Manchu sounds still more daunting. Finally, Borrow arranged in meticulous detail, and in spoken Russian, its printing by Russian workers.

Borrow's eloquence and persuasion were no less impressive than his linguistic skills and stamina. In Spain, he achieved what must be the salesman's ultimate accolade: by the conviction of his preaching, he got a number of customs officials who had been instructed to confiscate his illegal Bibles actually to buy them from him! Later, in the course of exploring the wilder regions of the Iberian peninsula, he came within a hair's breadth of public execution but, by means of good luck and skill, managed to walk away a free man.

After a charmed life of audacity, unspeakable hardship and danger in various countries, sprinkled with the eccentric drama that he so loved, Borrow retired to the calm of East Anglia to write his autobiography. Not surprisingly, he found life in the country to be somewhat lacking in adventure, and he yearned to be on the road again.

Michael Collie wrote of Borrow:

> 'One part of the young Borrow was gregarious, inquisitive, outward-going. He went to prize-fights, bear pits, taverns, galleries. He made many acquaintances, and *Lavengro* makes clear how much he enjoyed his first explorations in London. But another important part of this young man was essentially private, secretive, withdrawn, and these two parts of him were never reconciled, except in his books, creatively.'

Insights into obsessionality

In *Lavengro* Borrow wrote:

> 'With respect to my mind and its qualities I shall be more explicit; for were I to maintain much reserve on this point, many things which appear in these memoirs would be highly mysterious to the reader, indeed incomprehensible. Perhaps no two individuals were ever more unlike in mind and disposition than my brother and myself: as light is opposed to darkness, so was that happy, brilliant, cheerful child to the sad and melancholy being who sprang from the same stock as himself; and was nurtured by the same milk.

'A lover of nooks and retired corners, I was as a child in the habit of fleeing from society, and of sitting for hours together with my head on my breast. What I was thinking about it would be difficult to say at this distance of time; I remember perfectly well, however, being ever conscious of a peculiar heaviness within me, and at times of a strange sensation of fear, which occasionally amounted to horror, and for which I could assign no real cause whatever.'

As a young man, Borrow spent time in rumination about the meaning of existence and truth. His agonies, aroused by appreciation of the transient nature of existence, have been vividly recorded. In *Lavengro* he wrote:

'Then there was myself; for what was I born? Are not all things to be forgotten? That's incomprehensible: yet is it not so? Those butterflies fall and are forgotten. In what is man better than a butterfly? All then is born to be forgotten. Ah! that was a pang indeed . . .

'In truth, it was a sore vexation of spirit to me when I saw, as the wise men saw of old, that whatever I could hope to perform must necessarily be of very temporary duration; and, if so, why do it? I said to myself, whatever name I can acquire, will it endure for eternity? Scarcely so.'

Later in *Lavengro* he described a specific rumination:

'My own peculiar ideas with respect to everything being a lying dream began also to revive. Sometimes at midnight, after having toiled for hours at my occupations, I would fling myself back on my chair, look about the poor apartment, dimly lighted by an unsnuffed candle, or upon the heaps of books and papers before me, and exclaim – "Do I exist? Do these things, which I see about me, exist or do they not?"'

In an account that undoubtedly speaks from personal experience, Borrow beautifully described an antagonism between thoughts of opposite polarity:

'No one is fortunate unless he is happy, and it is impossible for a being constructed like myself to be happy for an hour, or even enjoy peace and tranquillity; most of our pleasures and pains are the effects of imagination, and wherever the sensibility is great, the imagination is great also. No sooner has my imagination raised up an image of pleasure, than it is sure to conjure up one of distress and gloom; these two antagonistic ideas instantly commence a struggle in my mind, and the gloomy one generally, I may say, invariably, prevails.'

Thus, for example, Borrow was able to turn the pleasure of a gift into pain, by doubting the ownership of the gift.

Compulsions

An obsessive compulsive problem is described in *Lavengro*, where Borrow related to the time when his mother was taken ill:

'. . . the thought that I might possibly lose her now rushed into my mind for the first time; it was terrible, and caused me unspeakable misery, I may say horror.

'Suddenly I found myself doing that which even at the time struck me as being highly singular; I found myself touching particular objects that were near me, and to which my fingers seemed to be attracted by an irresistible impulse. It was now the table or the chair that I was compelled to touch; now the bell-rope; now the handle of the door; now I would touch the wall; and the next moment, stooping down, I would place the point of my finger upon the floor: and so I continued to do day after day; frequently I would struggle to resist the impulse, but invariably in vain. I have even rushed away from the object, but I was sure to return, the impulse was too strong to be resisted: I quickly hurried back, compelled by the feeling within me to touch the object. Now I need not tell you that what impelled me to these actions was the desire to prevent my mother's death; whenever I touched any particular object, it was with a view to baffling the evil chance, as you would call it – in this instance my mother's death.'

In his *The Life of George Borrow*, Herbert Jenkins quoted an observation made to him by a Mr Watts-Dunton:

'There was nothing that Borrow strove against with more energy than the curious impulse, which he seems to have shared with Dr Johnson, to touch objects along his path in order to save himself from the evil chance. He never conquered the superstition. In walking through Richmond Park he would step out of his way constantly to touch a tree, and he was offended if the friend he was with seemed to observe it.'

Another compulsive ritual that Borrow described in the context of preventing evil happenings was to climb an elm tree next to his house and touch the top branch.

'... the difficulty and peril of such a feat startled me; I reasoned against the feeling, and strove more strenuously than I had ever done before; I even made a solemn vow not to give way to the temptation, but I believe nothing less than chains, and those strong ones, could have restrained me.'

Then Borrow gave a beautiful account of the dilemma of the obsessional:

'Indeed, all the time that I was performing these strange feats, I knew them to be highly absurd, yet the impulse to perform them was irresistible – a mysterious dread hanging over me till I had given way to it; even at that early period I frequently used to reason within myself as to what could be the cause of my propensity to touch, but of course I could come to no satisfactory conclusion respecting it; being heartily ashamed of the practice, I never spoke of it to anyone, and was at all times highly solicitous that no one should observe my weakness.'

Agonies of perfectionism are richly described in *Lavengro*. The reaction of an author following a good reception of his first published work formed the subject in this case:

'... the reception which it met with was far beyond my wildest expectations. The public were delighted with it, but what were my feelings? Anything, alas! but those of delight. No sooner did the public express its satisfaction at the result of my endeavours, than my perverse imagination began to conceive a thousand chimerical doubts...

'... I forthwith commenced touching the objects around me, in order to baffle the evil chance, as you call it; it was neither more nor less than a doubt of the legality of my claim to the thoughts, expressions, and situations contained in the book; that is, to all that constituted the book.'

Reflections

Later *Lavengro* describes the fear of death and what might follow it, in a way that would doubtless vividly ring true for anyone who has this type of obsessional rumination:

' – and how long could I hope to live? perhaps fifty years; at the end of which I must go to my place; and then I would count the months and the days, nay even the hours which yet intervened between me and my doom. Sometimes I would comfort myself with the idea that a long time would elapse before my time would be out; but then again I thought that, however long the term might be, it must be out at last; and then I would fall into an agony, during which I would almost wish that the term were out, and that I were in my place; the horrors of which I thought could scarcely be worse than what I then endured.'

Analysis

Reading Borrow is a considerable challenge, requiring some detective work because he manages to combine fact, fiction and fantasy into a uniquely confusing blend even in what seems to be autobiographical material. We can speculate that Borrow met some very articulate obsessionals in the course of his travels, or that he simply invented the characters and their problems, or, as seems much more likely, he wove his own obsessional experiences into the characters he describes. There is likely to have been a relatively low probability of finding by chance 'out-of-the-closet' obsessive-compulsives in 19th-century rural England. Therefore the first possibility defies statistical expectation, even for someone meeting as many people as Borrow. The second is implausible in our view, because the accounts are far too good to be the product of invention and Borrow was not a noted inventor.

In the second volume of his autobiography, entitled *The Romany Rye*, Borrow reveals more interesting information relevant to the present study, as well as extolling his own virtues at some length. He returns to consider the rich gentleman in *Lavengro* who has the touching compulsion, and asks if 'the kindness and providence of God' are not revealed in his case. 'This being has great gifts and many amiable qualities but does not everybody see that his besetting sin is selfishness?' The obsessional behaviour is seen as a way of curing the man of his egoism.

Hans Christian Andersen (1805–1875)

Childhood

Hans Christian Andersen was born to poor parents in Odense, Denmark, in 1805. Fortunately, because of Andersen's enthusiasm for writing everything down, not least that which concerned himself, a mountain of material was left for posterity. Hans Christian was born into a family in which folklore, magic, superstition and rituals played an ever-present role. Death omens, ghosts and fortune-telling were much in evidence. The morbid, dramatic and romantic were to hold a life-long fascination for him. Somewhat predictably, he was scared of the dark and frightened to walk past a churchyard. Sometimes the young boy was sent on an errand that involved passing a demolished convent. This place was considered haunted; it seemed to emit a strange light but, believing that spirits cannot cross water, he felt safe when he reached the far side of the river. Hans Christian's father, who was devoted to his son, suffered from occasional depression and was prone to spells of silent rumination.

In 1811, when Hans Christian was six, the Great Comet appeared in the sky. His own life-story records that he believed the superstition regarding the destruction of Earth that would be caused by the comet. 'I expected every moment that the comet would rush down, and the day of judgement would come.' A belief in divine providence over his own life was something that accompanied Andersen for all of his days.

Odense jail and lunatic asylum, both of which he visited, held an irresistible mixture of terror and fascination for the young Hans Christian. His mother and grandmother spoilt him, protected him and instilled in him the belief that he was somewhat different from other children – a natural genius. Hans Christian didn't play with other children, and was regarded as very odd and prudish. He preferred the company of his toys and puppets, his dolls and books. Some time was devoted to praying. He would spend hours in the garden inside a tent improvised from his mother's apron, engaged in making dresses for the dolls, or just ruminating.

> 'I was a singularly dreamy child, and so constantly went about with my eyes shut, as at last to give the impression of having weak sight, although the sense of sight was especially cultivated by me.'

Andersen opened his autobiography with 'There is a loving God, who directs all things for the best.' None the less, in Andersen's belief system it was worth keeping God informed of one's wishes. His auto-biography shows his wish to test the control of destiny, a factor of much interest to students of the obsessional personality. After being told about the omniscient and omnipotent nature of God, he recorded:

> 'That idea occupied my whole mind, and towards evening, as I went alone from the court, where there was a deep pond, and stood upon some stones which were just within the water, the thought passed through my head whether God actually knew every thing which was to happen there. Yes, he has now determined that I should live and be so many years old, thought I; but, if I now were to jump into the water here and drown myself, then it would not be as he wished; and all at once I was firmly and resolutely determined to drown myself: I ran to where the water was deepest, and then a new thought passed through my soul. "It is the devil who wishes to have power over me!" I uttered a loud cry, and, running away from the place as if I were pursued, fell weeping into my mother's arms.'

(Similar childhood testings of God were recorded in John Bunyan's *Autobiography of a Soul* and Jean-Jacques Rousseau's *Confessions*.)

Hans Christian was drawn to the theatre, and tried writing and per-forming plays, using his parents as an audience. The child loved the limelight that these plays and his fine singing voice provided. Acting became such an 'obsession' that his parents were led to wonder whether their much-loved son was mad. The plays often had morbid and macabre themes, one being an adaptation of *Hamlet*. Being told that royalty probably addressed each other in foreign tongues, he devised a hybrid language for the royal parts. In one, a princess greets her father, the king, with the original, if somewhat inelegant 'Guten Morgen, mon père! Har De godt sleeping?'

Hans Christian's mother wanted him to become a tailor or book-binder, but his ambition was to be an actor. Overwhelming egocentricity and self-confidence would not permit a humble job; he craved public recognition. The boy protested to his mother that he had read stories of many men from humble origins who went on to better things.

When he was 14, Hans Christian's mother waved him off on the mail-coach for Copenhagen, where he was determined to seek his for-tune. When the boat arrived at Zealand, his reaction was to fall down on his knees and pray for God's help. After some tears and further prayers on the way, he finally arrived at the big city.

Copenhagen

Life was to be far from easy. Naïve and trusting but driven by an overwhelming ambition, he encountered numerous frustrations and hardships. He found a tiny room but could not raise enough money for the deposit. Hans Christian's reaction on finding himself alone in the room of this potential landlady shows an affinity for superstition.

> '. . . I seated myself on the sofa, and contemplated the portrait of her deceased husband. I was so wholly a child that as the tears rolled down my cheeks I wetted the eyes of the portrait with my tears, in order that the dead man might feel how troubled I was, and influence the heart of his wife. She must have seen that nothing more was to be drained out of me, for when she returned to the room she said she would receive me into her house for the sixteen rix dollars. I thanked God and the dead man.'

Still, life was tough. Andersen was very clumsy in his movements, somewhat weird in looks and often treated as a joke by Copenhageners. However, he could not face the humiliation of returning to Odense. Suicide, though seriously contemplated, was not an option, because it was a sin.

Throughout his life, literally from the moment of birth onwards, Andersen spent an inordinate amount of time in tears: tears of sorrow, of joy, of sentiment, of excitement, of awe for the singing of Jenny Lind, and occasionally of unambiguous manipulation. Regularly he prayed that things might get better, and, when they did, God was thanked. In the end, Hans Christian was admitted briefly to the ballet, his first appearance being as one of a group of trolls. His memoirs record:

> '. . . our names stood printed in the bill. That was a moment in my life, when my name was printed! I fancied I could see in it a nimbus of immortality. I was continually looking at the printed paper. I carried the programme of the ballet with me at night to bed, lay and read my name by candle-light – in short, I was happy.'

Andersen's talents were to move from the ballet to that of writing stories and poems, for which he was soon to be famous throughout Denmark, and ultimately the world.

Insights into obsessionality

He had a genius for inventing situations of fear and seemed to have been as afraid of hypothetical and highly improbable events as of immediate real danger. He had an obsession about dying from drowning or fire or as the victim of murder. His fear of seduction, robbery, dogs and losing his passport seemed to be carried with him wherever he went. He also suffered from agoraphobia, being unable to cross a large crowded square without an escort.

Considering such a daunting list of dangers, one might have supposed that Andersen would have spent his life in the relative safety of a house, but nothing could be further from the truth. Not only did he never have a home of his own, preferring to stay with friends or in hotels, but his autobiography describes the life of a fanatical traveller, constantly on the move and meeting people in Sweden, France, England, Italy and Holland. Even in unambiguously dangerous situations, after much ruminating, curiosity was sometimes able to dominate over caution. Some obsessionals are nothing if not stubborn and determined!

We can gain an impression of the thoughts that troubled Andersen for so much of his life from the following entry in his diary, concerning the Franco-Prussian war in 1870:

'The war in France overwhelms me, I am suffering from *idées fixes* which make me mad; the terrors of France are constantly showing themselves before me as if I had to live through them myself: I see myself pierced by bayonets, the city is burning, friends are dying, or I dream of being thrown into prison.'

Andersen was a man of high moral standards, prudish and a bachelor. He probably never had any sexual experience, though he recorded fascination with prostitutes he saw in Naples, as if torn between approach and avoidance. Wolfgang Lederer has described him as 'Forever an "applicant", forever insistently ingratiating, but never frankly asserting himself.' He was essentially a loner despite being known by a vast circle of contacts throughout most of Europe, kings and queens, composers and writers, from whom he endlessly solicited praise and appreciation of his own fame.

His life was a textbook case of obsessional rumination: something he had just eaten would poison him, he would miss an important connection unless he arrived very early, he would be returned to poverty;

some trivial event would be blown up out of all proportion and be seen as leading to his death.

A process of competition between thoughts is recorded by a friend, William Bloch, describing a visit to Vienna:

'Andersen was choking and had to leave the table, accompanied by our host and hostess, and everything was very quiet while Andersen was heard coughing and spitting in the other room. Against the protest of the hostess he maintained that there had been a pin in the meat; he had swallowed it and could clearly feel it sitting inside him. That evening and the following day he was very worried about the consequences. His anxiety was so pronounced that it had completely removed his fear that a little spot above one of his eyebrows might grow into a large excrescence which would cover the eye, which again had made him forget that he might rupture himself because I had touched his stomach slightly with my walking stick, which again made him abandon the thought of having hydrarthrosis of the knee ['water on the knee'], something he was much concerned about when he arrived in Vienna.'

Andersen was able to ruin an evening out by imagining that he had forgotten to lock the front door. In the course of a night he needed repeatedly to rise in order to check that he really had extinguished the candle by his bed, though he never failed to do this very carefully on retiring. When sending letters, he would worry that he had mixed up envelopes. On one occasion, having written to King George of Greece, he became obsessed that he had written 'Otto' instead of 'George'. Another obsession was that he had paid the wrong amount of money in a shop.

The dark side of Andersen's personality emerges very clearly in his autobiography, and these writings are of importance in the study of the obsessional personality.

'At the end of October, 1845, I left Copenhagen. Formerly I had thought when I set out on a journey, God! what wilt thou permit to happen to me on this journey! This time my thoughts were, God, what will happen to my friends at home during this long time! And I felt a real anxiety. In one year the hearse may drive up to the door many times, and whose name may shine upon the coffin! The proverb says, when one suddenly feels a cold shudder, "now death passes over my grave". The shudder is still colder when the thoughts pass over the graves of our best friends.'

The theme of avoiding harm appears in many of Andersen's obsessions, even though the logic that might lead to harm would seem to be somewhat convoluted. For example, he was once given a banknote in his change in a restaurant in Frankfurt, and later discovered that the note was no longer legal tender. He described this later in a letter to a friend in Frankfurt, and posted the letter, only to find himself occupied with the thought that it could lead to the waiter being fired. So he returned to the post office and retrieved the letter.

To use Andersen's own expression, he was able to 'plague himself to the most exquisite degree'. He wrote this in his diary on the day in which he paid a visit to the tailor's to collect a coat. On finding his coat was not ready, the tailor lent him another. This troubled Andersen, because he was afraid that the coat might belong to someone else. The person might come up and say 'You're wearing my coat!'

He noted that the essence of his creative work consisted of allowing his imagination to flow but that this same imagination was the source of much inconvenience:

> 'I possessed a peculiar talent, that of lingering on the gloomy side of life, of extracting the bitter from it, and tasting it; and understood well, when the whole was exhausted, how to torment myself.
>
> 'I betrayed more and more in my writings an unhealthy turn of mind. I felt an inclination to seek for the melancholy in life, and to linger on the dark side of things; I became sensitive, and thought rather of the blame than the praise which was lavished on me.'

However, the melancholy needs to be put into context; Andersen also vividly recorded moments of immense joy in his life.

Andersen took action to pre-empt the danger contained in his fears. For instance, just in case there was a fire, he carried a rope in his trunk so that he would be able to descend from the window. Somewhat more bizarre was his fear of being buried alive, and to prevent this he would leave a note by his bed with 'Jeg er skindød' written on it (meaning 'I only seem to be dead', or 'I am in suspended animation'). He repeatedly requested friends to promise to cut an artery before sealing his coffin. Andersen's ability to allow the anticipation of disaster to detract from the pleasures of good things to come is illustrated by when he was given the freedom of Odense, the realisation of a fortune-teller's prediction. He predicted that someone would spoil the big event, possibly by trying to murder him.

Literary fame also seems to have set the scene for ruminations and self-doubt, a craving for perfection, as his autobiography reveals:

> 'There is something elevating, but at the same time something terrific, in seeing one's thoughts spread so far, and among so many people; it is, indeed, almost a fearful thing to belong to so many. The noble and the good in us become a blessing; but the bad, one's errors, shoot forth also, and involuntarily the thought forces itself from us: God! let me never write down a word of which I shall not be able to give an account to Thee. A peculiar feeling, a mixture of joy and anxiety, fills my heart every time my good genius conveys my fictions to a foreign people.'

Fear of oblivion is evident in the following diary entry, made on 5 March 1872 and prompted by the death of a friend:

> 'Is he now dust and ashes, dead, extinguished, put out like a flame which does not exist any more? O God, my Lord! Can you let us disappear completely? I have a fear of that, and I have become too clever and unhappy.'

Charles Darwin (1809–1882)

Charles Darwin is the founder of the theory of evolution – that, over millions of years, the species of animal in existence today, including humans, have gradually evolved from simpler forms. The influential American philosopher, Daniel Dennett, described this as 'the best idea that anyone has ever had . . . ahead of Newton and Einstein and everyone else'. Darwin discovered not only the principles of natural selection (that animals are, in effect, tested for their suitability for their environment and thereby evolve to fit it) but also mechanisms of plant fertilisation, formation of coral reefs and others.

It is sad to reflect that a mind able to create thoughts of such very special and profound significance was also exquisitely tuned to produce others of a very black and unwanted kind. Darwin suffered from various disorders of a neurotic kind, including psychosomatic illness (the type in which neurotic states are associated with disturbance in the body, such as stomach upset and skin rashes). Obsessionality seemed to be a feature of these.

Charles Darwin's grandfather Erasmus Darwin – a poet, physician and naturalist – was an inspiration to Charles in terms of his studying medicine and postulating evolutionary theory. After completing his degree in medicine from Edinburgh University and theology from Cambridge University, Charles Darwin embarked on a world-surveying voyage on board HMS *Beagle* (1831–1836). The evidence he collected and the observations he made during this scientific trip subsequently led to the theory of evolution and modification of species, which he published in 1859.

Childhood

In his early years, Darwin was a friendly and gregarious young man and, according to his own recollection, was of excellent health. However, there were two main problems as remembered by his brother and sister. First, Charles was susceptible to psychosomatic ill health: when confronted with unpleasant news he tended to be extremely disturbed and have an upset stomach, which could last several days. Second, he had what he described as 'a disturbance' of the hands, a lip 'affliction' and a disease of the skin, which, expressed in Darwin's own words, could have been the result of his 'manner of living'. All these manifestations made him feel ashamed and depressed, and this eased only when his environment changed.

The voyage of the Beagle and its significance

In 1831, Darwin was due to sail around the world on board HMS *Beagle*. This year was particularly bad for his health. He was under considerable pressure because his father disapproved of this journey and the departure of the *Beagle* was postponed several times due to weather conditions. On top of this, Darwin was worried about the possibility of contracting infectious diseases during the trip, about his seasickness and about the smallness of his cabin. However, his main anxiety was caused by the fear that he would become unable to work. These anxieties caused palpitations, a 'lip problem', stomach upset, vomiting and depression, which ceased on board the *Beagle* (from December 1831 to October 1836).

During the first year after his return to England, Darwin was kept busy writing scientific papers about the geological and zoological data that he collected on his *Beagle* travels. These papers were generally accepted and, what was more important, he had almost no health complaints. However, by 1838 Darwin was agonising over his evolution theory; as a result the stomach pain reappeared, followed by palpitations. He obviously connected his anxieties with the theory, as he wrote in his evolution notebooks, that his imagination influenced his body actions.

Emma

In 1839, Charles married his cousin Emma Wedgwood (of the famous pottery family). Emma would be Darwin's support and nurse for the rest of his life. Charles deeply loved Emma and seemed to be happy. But a deep-rooted conflict in their relationship was the cause of growing anxieties. Emma was a very religious person and suffered because her husband did not always share her staunch beliefs. Rightly or wrongly, Darwin's principal work – his theory of evolution – undermined Emma's religious faith. Thus, from the very beginning of married life, Darwin developed anxieties about the conflict between his family and his work, about the theory of evolution itself and about Emma's health and well-being.

In the early years of the marriage, the psychosomatic manifestations worsened. Now, after talking to anybody other than immediate members of the family and one or two friends, Darwin 'almost always' experienced 'excitement, violent shivering and vomiting attacks'. It could be that he did not like to be interrupted from his work or did not feel comfortable to discuss and reveal his scientific thoughts, or both. Whatever the reason, Darwin started to avoid people; when relatives visited him, he would sit silently after dinner for some time simply to keep them company.

Things get worse

In 1848, Darwin's father, Robert, aged 82, was seriously ill, had difficulties in breathing and had a 'dying sensation'. Soon after this, Charles Darwin experienced 'almost continual anxiety', suffered from violent vomiting, trembling hands and visual disturbances, and feared that he was 'rapidly' dying. In fact, he was so scared of death and of losing his father that, when his father died, he did not attend the funeral and refused to be one of his executors. This severe attack of illness continued for several months after his father's death. The severity was such that Charles avoided everyone, even his sisters, when they visited him. He consulted a doctor, who classified his illness as 'unique'. As an index of his anxiety over death, Darwin did not attend the funeral of his beloved daughter Annie, and never visited her grave.

Darwin started his self-observation, making daily entries in his 'Diary of Health'. He made entries for more than five years, from 1849 to 1855. The diary reveals the manifestations of his illness and his own thoughts about it.

Obsessional thoughts

Darwin wrote about his various obsessional thoughts and how he could not get away from them. Being a workaholic, hard work was one solution. In a letter to his friend Hooker, Darwin talked about nocturnal obsessional thoughts: 'I could not sleep and whatever I did in the day haunted me at night with vivid and most wearing repetition.' These were agonising thoughts about the theory of evolution, fear of humiliation about it, fear that his children would inherit his kind of illness and fear of death. The thoughts, as he himself put it, were 'of horrid spectacle', and to stop them he would try 'closing his eyes firmly' but they would not go away. The bad thoughts during the night were more persistent than those in the day, because at night he was not distracted from them by activity.

Darwin craved reassurance from others, being 'pathologically' modest and self-critical and with a quite overbearing conscience. He felt himself to be ugly, and the recognition of even a modest dose of vanity in himself was a source of distress. Darwin found that one means of easing nagging doubts was the repetition to himself hundreds of times the mantra: 'I have worked as hard as I could, and no man can do more than this'. He was often obsessed with the idea that he might have been misunderstood and this prevented him from sleeping. For example, after a discussion of a matter of no great significance with the vicar of Downe, Darwin returned in the night to the vicar's home to check that the wrong impression had not been created.

More than 20 agonising years passed after Darwin returned from the *Beagle* voyage. In these years he spent time systematising, classifying, writing and rewriting the drafts of the theory of evolution. Alas, at the same time, he described himself as 'the most stupid Dog in all England' (thereby reminding us of just how wrong obsessionals can be when it comes to self-assessment!). He referred to his work as 'imperfect and with many mistakes' and had tortuous thoughts that it was immoral and irreligious.

The origin of the species

Finally, in November 1859, after correcting several proofs, his book – *The Origin of Species* – was published. By December Darwin started to receive letters expressing various opinions on his theory. Some of his friends admired him and his revolutionary ideas, but some ridiculed, disapproved of his theory and called him 'the most dangerous man in England'. All of this caused anxiety and as a result Darwin suffered painfully. In one of his letters, he expressed tremendous happiness at having passed 52 hours (!) without vomiting. At about this time Darwin wrote his famous quote about his illness: 'I know well that my head would have failed years ago, had not my stomach always saved me . . .' He realised the connection between his mind and physical manifestations. This realisation came at an early age, even before the *Beagle* voyage. Darwin made the connection between, on the one hand, the physical manifestations of his illness, lack of energy and stress of mental conflict and, on the other, disagreement with the views of people he respected. Even more so, he probably understood that his stomach pain, vomiting etc. were caused by his mind and, ironically enough, they distracted him, at least partly, from his obsessional thoughts.

Sometimes Darwin even expressed gratitude that he had eczema, because it saved him 'from distractions of society and amusement'. During 1837–1839 he experienced only mild manifestations of his psychosomatic disorders; as a result, these were the most productive years of his life, the years when he pioneered his evolutionary theory and socialised. Then, in the mid-1800s, his state was so bad that it nearly destroyed him. Darwin himself estimated that he lost several years – indeed, the best of his working life. Throughout his life he tried to make the best of what he had, and struggled against the devastating and killing effects of his illness.

His desire to work was his driving force, managing the 'worst states' and regaining the will. 'I would sooner be the wretched contemptible invalid, which I am, than live the life of an idle squire', he wrote after two periods of 'worst states' and having inherited the money from his father, which allowed him to relax and work less. He always spoke about his work as the only thing that made his life bearable.

The Sandwalk

In 1842 Darwin's house-hunting for his family finally achieved success: he found a suitable house in the village of Down, Kent. The routine of Darwin's life at Down was like clockwork. In 1846 he rented a strip of land, which he planted with shrubs and trees and erected a fence. There he chose and carefully marked a quarter mile of path that he called 'the Sandwalk'. He walked this route obsessionally every day, with total disregard to any circumstances in or outside the family. His daughter Annie and, later, the boys and sometimes visitors such as Huxley joined Darwin on the Sandwalk. His daily schedule never altered: breakfast, work, reading letters, Sandwalk pace, lunch, responding to letters, nap, work, rest, tea, listening to Emma reading books and finally bed. Even in his last year (1882), Darwin still performed his daily ritualistic routine of pacing the Sandwalk, though the pace was slower and the laps were fewer.

The Sandwalk was doubtless a welcome means by which to gain physical exercise, and such a routine might have been expected to contribute to his physical and mental efficiency. However, the rigorous, rigid persistence with the same path over and over again for nearly 36 years could point to a more obsessive nature and meaning of the walk. Surely he could have varied the route somewhat for country walking!

Things get better

The last decade of Darwin's life (1872–1882) was accompanied by less pain and suffering. One might ask why it is that the illness, although of long-standing and still occurring in acute bouts, eased by the end of his life. Indeed, Emma and their servant observed that Darwin's overall health had improved. He still suffered from anxiety but complained less about the stomach pain, vomiting and palpitations. The amelioration of old and chronic illness could have several reasons. First, by this time, Darwin had stopped writing about controversial issues and tried to avoid emotional involvement when discussing them. Secondly, he was doing scientific research on plants, which he found very healing during the years of furious debates over *The Origin*. Of course, his botanical investigations were causing him anxieties and mental stress but their basis was not associated with considerations of 'immorality' and 'heresy' as there were with the theory of evolution. Moreover, during this time his theory became accepted by his peers, friends and people whose opinion he valued. His financial state greatly improved from investments, his property and books. Finally, although Darwin worried much about the inheritance aspect of his illness, his children gave him much happiness. They grew up, got married and had successful careers.

Inheritance?

Emma Darwin gave birth to ten children, seven of whom survived and lived long lives (sadly, two died young from natural causes). Five of the surviving children developed hypochondriasis, which could have had any of several causes. All of them had long childhood illnesses and were aware of their father's illness, his frequent observation of their pulse and his conviction that the illness was passed through to other generations. One particular daughter – Henrietta, known in the literature on Darwin as Aunt Etty – caused her parents anxiety from childhood. As Darwin's granddaughter, Gwen Raverat, remembered, when Aunt Etty was 13 years old, she was told by her doctor to take breakfast in bed, because of a 'low fever'. She lived in morbid fear of illness following the death of her sister Annie. Needless to say, Aunt Etty never in her life had her breakfast otherwise, although she lived until she was 86.

All his life, Darwin was troubled by his illnesses, tried to understand them, and meticulously recorded anything that had an impact on his health.

In *The Variation of Animals and Plants under Domestication*, Darwin discussed inheritance. He gave the example of a boy, known to him personally, who had a very peculiar habit. When excited, the boy would raise his hands to eye level, while moving his fingers. Darwin reported that even when an old man 'the boy' could not resist this habit. He grew up to father eight children, and one of his daughters had a similar strange habit. What makes this observation of Darwin particularly interesting is the strong possibility that in reality Darwin was talking about himself. Darwin was extremely anxious about 'transmitting' his disease to his own children (also eight in number).

Reflections on Darwin's life

Five years after Darwin's death, Francis Darwin published his father's *Life and Letters*. In these Charles described his illness and made the

connection between tortuous obsessional thoughts (related and unrelated to his work) and the severity of physical symptoms. His heroic
and stoical nature is admirable and his persistence in trying to understand more about the laws of nature is commendable. By rigidly
constructing his daily routine (another exhibition of the obsessional
trait), working intensively during the 'good' periods, Darwin managed
to produce an extraordinary amount of work and to achieve tri-
umphant glory despite a delicate psychological nature, severe anxieties
and obsessional thoughts.

Freudian explanation of Darwin's illness?

We are not drawn to Freudian explanations. However, Darwin has been
a favourite subject for speculation by analysts of the Freudian persuasion. It might be argued that Freud's analysis of psychological problems
was generally based on a reflection of his own problems. At the root of
his explanation of Darwin's condition lies the so-called 'Oedipus complex' (an association is formed between erotic sensations at the genitals
and sexual fantasy images, i.e. a boy experiencing sexual desire towards
his mother; this sets up a conflict in which the boy is envious of his
father's sexuality and the latter's access to his mother). Freudian analysts saw Darwin's illness as a reaction against his father; the *Beagle*
trip was an escape from his father, so the anxieties eased during the
voyage. After returning from the trip, the anxieties came back because
of religious conflict with the concept of the Creator, i.e. his father. To
add to this, Darwin's marriage represented the annihilation of his
father and his own status as a sexual partner of his mother. This
hypothesis lacks any sort of scientific proof.

John Bowlby and Darwin

The English psychiatrist John Bowlby presented an analysis of Darwin.
Although influenced by Freudian ideas and giving weight to the death
of Darwin's mother, the analysis took a distinctly different line of argument from that just given. It is one that Bowlby was able to support
with some scientific evidence. He attributed Darwin's troubles to his
failure to mourn properly the passing of his mother. Bowlby cited evidence pointing to the stiff and unemotional family environment, which
encouraged the young Darwin to suppress emotional reaction ('sealing
in silence'). Bowlby's line of argument is that normal mourning allows

an adaptive readjustment to the changed circumstances. Darwin's response, rather than avoiding trauma, triggered the unconscious mind to store a memory of the event, which influenced subsequent psychological life. According to Bowlby, the suppressed event also has a profound effect upon the body such as to disrupt the heart and breathing (e.g. panic attacks).

Gioacchino Rossini (1792–1868)

In some respects, the Italian composer Gioacchino Rossini might seem to be an unlikely candidate for inclusion here. Handsome, generous, kind, charming, humorous and charismatic, superficially at least there is little to suggest an obsessional personality type. He appeared to have enjoyed to the full the good life of wine, women and song, possessing what the biographer of great musicians, Harold Schonberg, described as a 'happy-go-lucky temperament'. Furthermore, Rossini's musical creation is characterised by its ability to trigger pure pleasure. Also, quite unlike some of the other heroes of this chapter, he did not earn a universal reputation as an obsessional perfectionist. Indeed, in spite of his prodigious output, some have described him as lazy and willing to cut corners. He would often leave things to the last minute before getting down to serious composition, even writing the overture to an opera on the same day as its first performance.

However, Rossini serves to remind us of the often-contradictory aspects within personality and disorder. He is reported to have told a friend: 'I have all of women's ills. All that I lack is the uterus.' There are indications of obsessional features in Rossini's make-up and signs that he was troubled by obsessional thoughts. His biographer Francis Toye describes him as 'timid' and 'highly neurotic'. Some have speculatively diagnosed manic–depressive illness (an alternating rhythm of high and low mood) but this is not incompatible with obsessionality.

The young man

Rossini was born on 29 February 1792 in Pesaro, a port on Italy's Adriatic coast. He displayed an enormous musical talent as a child, being able to sing in opera and play the piano, violin and viola. However, he also earned an early reputation for high spirits and getting into mischief. Francis Toye writes: 'There can be no doubt that for sheer naughtiness Rossini's boyhood is unparalleled in the annals of the great masters of music.'

While still a teenager, his talent as a composer was becoming evident. By the age of 21, Rossini had achieved world fame.

The composer

At the height of his fame, Rossini was idolised and courted throughout Europe. He and his wife were much sought after as guests at parties, and their own hospitality at musical evenings was legendary. Then suddenly at the age of 37, soon after his greatest success, the opera *William Tell*, Rossini announced his retirement.

The reasons for this decision have provided a favourite topic for speculation among music historians. Some have cited an intrinsic laziness, combined with the acquisition of enormous wealth. Others cite a conservative disapproval with the direction that the world of music was taking. Still others have pointed to his medical troubles: chronic gonorrhoea, hypochondria and insomnia.

Obsessional personality?

Much of Rossini's personality would stand in stark contrast to the traits often described as 'obsessional'. However, psychological life is rarely simple; people can possess a complex mixture of traits, and Rossini's contemporaries noted certain obsessional features of his lifestyle, such as extreme emotional sensitivity.

According to the English psychiatrist Anthony Storr, Rossini's ritualistic behaviour manifested itself in similar ways to that of his fellow composers Haydn and Stravinsky. They were preoccupied with cleanliness and order. They rose early, worked regularly and kept to a timetable of activity. Rossini's wigs were arranged in meticulous order. The furniture in the study was arranged symmetrically and the objects around Rossini were placed in symmetrical order. When not working 'at the last minute', Rossini constantly perfected his compositions; even when copying them out he made changes, trying to perfect them. The order and neatness of his study were striking, and it was difficult to associate this room with an artistic personality, rightly or wrongly usually characterised by disorder.

Obsessional disorder?

A hint of OCD is suggested. Francis Toye records that after a friend had been killed in a fire, Rossini's 'morbid imagination, his hypersensitive nerves, gave him no rest; he was, one of his biographers tells us, prostrate for many days'.

Toye also argues that 'brilliant wit was to be a mask for profound depression'. As a different shade of emphasis, one might speculate that Rossini hit on the medicine of humour for treating emotional disturbances.

Rossini refused to live in a house heated by gas for fear of an explosion. When on a visit to Belgium, he decided to try out the latest invention, the railway, escaping incognito to Antwerp. The experience, although by any objective standards amounting to a perfectly normal journey, caused him to faint and left his nerves shattered such that he was ill for some days afterwards. (Thank God that he didn't have to commute into London in the 21st century!) Rossini was never again able to get into a train. Paradoxically, this probably greatly increased his danger, as the only alternative was that of traversing snow-bound Europe in a horse-drawn coach.

When Rossini's father died, the son could not bear to look at the house again and immediately put it on the market.

At one point in his life in Paris, Rossini suffered from particular intrusions of sounds repeating themselves in his head. These were triggered by sounds in his environment. So much distress was caused to Rossini by this intrusion that his wife gave their porter a special fund to be used to bribe street musicians to keep away from the vicinity of their apartment.

Rather than being entirely arbitrary, certain of Rossini's particular obsessional thoughts make some sense in the context of his life and culture. For example, he is reported to have experienced extremes of guilt and shame about his venereal disease. He suffered moods of black despair and was obsessed with thoughts of death. In later years, his physical health was not good and being confined to bed was a perfect setting for triggering such thoughts. He was obsessed that he might be forgotten or despised by the world but these thoughts were lifted as his health improved and he was able to mingle once again with his adoring fans.

Although Rossini lived for 39 years after his retirement, he never wrote another note for publication. He did write small instrumental and vocal pieces for his own amusement, the names of which (e.g. *Prelude Convulsif, Valse Torture*) are revealing. They were collected under one title *Peches de vieillesse* (sins of old age).

Rossini was always superstitious, right up to his death on Friday the 13th (November 1868).

Søren Kierkegaard (1813–1855)

Søren Kierkegaard, philosopher and theologian, was born in Copenhagen in 1813. Kierkegaard was eventually to be called the father of existential philosophy. Psychologically speaking, he might be described as a full-time depressive with a morbid preoccupation and a part-time obsessional. However, he seems to have stretched philosophical rumination to its limits. We can think of few better prescriptions for obtaining a feeling of depression and existential fear than to read either Kierkegaard himself (which is hard going) or the excellent biography by Josiah Thompson (much lighter). For example, one of Kierkegaard's better-known works, *Fear and Trembling*, is an analysis of the agony experienced by Abraham as he prepared to sacrifice Isaac.

Childhood

As a child, Søren had been called 'the strange one' by other children. He would wear the same formal costume to school each day, unlike the informality of his classmates. Essentially a loner, introverted and melancholic, he lived a cocooned existence, brought up under the strict control of a devout father, himself a chronic depressive. Obedience to father was the rule. Young Søren would spend hours with his spinning-top – lost in thought. The father had demanding standards concerning such things as exactly how to polish shoes and at what time it was no longer safe for Søren to go out. They would sometimes spend long periods walking up and down their room hand-in-hand, while the father described to the young Søren imaginary street scenes in Copenhagen that they were 'passing'.

Later, Søren's university tutor was to have been exasperated by his: '. . . irresistible urge to sophistry, to hair-splitting that comes out on all occasions'.

The philosopher and theologian

Kierkegaard's aim in life might be described as one of completion or accommodation – of finding a master key; to use his own words, '. . . to clarify and solve the riddle of life has been my constant wish'. To this end, he had an insatiable appetite for writing, performed while alone but sometimes in evening dress as if to be entertaining company. In the toil of writing, he was able to escape from some of his torments. Kierkegaard gives us vivid insight:

> 'So I fared forth into life – initiated into all possible enjoyment yet never really enjoying, but rather (this was my single pleasure with respect to the pain of melancholy) working to produce the appearance that I enjoyed. I was acquainted with all sorts of people, yet it never aroused my mind that in any of them I had a confidant . . .'

Jolly, witty, argumentative in company, enjoying good food and wine, and yet through it all so clearly the ruminative, the melancholic stares out:

> 'I have just now come from a party where I was its life and soul; witticisms streamed from my lips, everyone laughed and admired me, but I went away – yes, the dash should be as long as the radius of the earth's orbit – and wanted to shoot myself.'
>
> 'The whole of existence makes me anxious, from the smallest fly to the mystery of the Incarnation: everything is unintelligible to me, most of all myself. . . . I suffer as a human being can suffer in indescribable melancholy, which always has to do with my thinking about my own existence.'
>
> 'The terrible thing about the total spiritual incapacity from which I suffer is precisely that it is coupled with a consuming longing, a spiritual passion.'

He seems to have been tormented by guilt associated with the feeling that he had let his father down. In addition to endless philosophical ruminations, there is evidence of conventional obsessionality. Things in his room were maintained in meticulous order. He insisted that his servant, Anders, should always maintain the room temperature at exactly 13¾°C. He kept 50 cups and saucers in his cabinet, one set in each of 50 patterns. His guests were asked which set they wanted their coffee served in, and then required to justify their choice. When walking the streets of Copenhagen, he always kept to the shadows and would never step over a sunlit patch.

Kierkegaard's biographer, J Thompson, noted:

'. . . the ritual elements but also the studied regularity of the meals bouillon on 29 out of 31 days – point to a life that has withdrawn into an aesthetic cocoon. Protected from distractions and interruptions by his faithful Anders, his rooms kept a constant 13¾°C with just a trace of Eau de Cologne in the air, Kierkegaard succeeded in keeping that "infected" world he hated at a distance.'

There were moments of light relief in Kierkegaard's life. In fact, he was capable of displaying an impish sense of humour and wasn't past a cruel practical joke. The melancholic philosopher was surprisingly good with children; an accomplished story-teller, he could easily switch into a world of fantasy. In these and some other regards, there are close similarities with his even more famous fellow-countryman, Hans Christian Andersen, whom he would sometimes encounter in the street during his strolls around Copenhagen. Both seemed to have lived a large part of their lives in what is best described as daydreams.

Henrik Ibsen (1828–1906)

Henrik Ibsen, the Norwegian dramatist and poet, was a pioneer and revolutionary figure within social drama, having a tremendous impact on the development of the theatre. Philosophical and psychological issues were present throughout his work. Ibsen not only portrayed the social world with depth but also challenged some of its most basic assumptions.

He ruthlessly exposed what he saw as hypocrisy and, in so doing, shocked many people. His scalpel was taken to the dogmas of established religion, the façade of 'respectable middle-class life' and the role of women. In some ways, by his exploration of the mind, Ibsen might qualify for the description of 'founding psychologist'. In works such as *Brand* and *Peer Gynt*, the theme of men chasing life-long dreams and at the end discovering emptiness and loneliness was developed. Probably the most personal is *When We Dead Awaken*. The story of a successful sculptor without artistic fulfilment portrays morbid introspective thoughts characteristic of those of Ibsen himself.

There is little hard evidence to suggest that Ibsen suffered from any form of serious obsessional disorder, though accounts written during his life note 'nervous fever'. However, there were some personality traits of obsessionality present and pundits have found it interesting to relate these to his emotional life, work and enormous creativity.

Childhood and teenage years

Ibsen was born on 20 March 1828 in the small town of Skien on Norway's coast. From his later recollections, it would seem that he was somewhat over-protected as a child and readily suffered guilt. The terms 'withdrawn', 'shy' and 'self-important' were commonly used to describe the young Ibsen. As one of his earliest memories, he recalled being taken by his nursemaid to the top of a tower and being allowed to sit in an open window. In the street below, his mother fainted on seeing him there.

A friend recalled the young Ibsen telling him 'with a curious ardour that he and his wife, if he ever acquired one, would have to live on separate floors, see each other at meal-times, and not address each other as "Du"' (the familiar form of 'you', equivalent to the French 'tu').

Ibsen had characteristics associated with obsessional behaviour from an early age. He was extremely meticulous about his clothes, a spot of dirt on them throwing him into panic.

The writer

Rooms he lived in were virtually dust and dirt free. Ibsen compulsively destroyed and rewrote his works, the end-product being what to most might constitute a 'perfect' manuscript. A fruitless search for perfection is suggested by a report that Ibsen never tired of looking at himself in mirrors. He had an obsession about time and punctuality, arriving for any appointment much earlier than was required. His tidiness with money is almost legendary; he kept meticulous records of spending. An early reputation for obsessive attention to dress persisted with the adult Ibsen taking an hour or more to get dressed in the morning. However, at one stage in his life, Ibsen was occasionally to be seen in public in a way that earned him a 'worst-dressed' distinction among Rome's Norwegian community. Perfectionism accompanied by intolerance is indicated in a letter to a companion: 'all my life I have turned my back on my parents, on my whole family, because I could not bear to continue a relationship based on imperfect understanding'.

Writers have noted strong similarities between Ibsen and Kierkegaard (see earlier). Both were loners, 'creatures of habit', shy of intimacy and lacking much in the way of joy in their lives. Both staged intellectual revolts of a kind against the establishment. We also see echoes of Hans Christian Andersen (discussed earlier) in Ibsen's psychological make-up; for example, repetitive intrusions of impending disaster and a kind of chronic social discomfort. Ibsen read Kierkegaard and met Andersen. These three characters must surely vie for some of the top positions in any rating of the most famous Scandinavians of all time.

Ibsen seems to have been plagued by anxieties, any one of which could have tipped over into a full-blown obsessional disorder. A companion noted: 'He had a curious fear of anything that might bring death or misadventure. This fear was not grounded in the thought of losing his life, but in a terror lest he might not achieve the artistic goal he had set himself.'

Analyses

On various fronts, Ibsen has formed a particularly irresistible topic of speculation. Both during his life and since, attempts have been made to identify Ibsen with his own characters, and a number of people in his personal circle identified themselves with his roles. As a writer on psychological themes, Ibsen has been a favourite subject among psychologists and psychoanalysts. One is drawn to look into the paradoxes – how could someone have such brilliant insight into the emotional plight of others and yet be apparently so emotionally remote? How could one who did so much to challenge conventionality insist on such rigid respect for protocol and formality in his dealings with others? Ibsen's biographer Michael Meyer suggested that Ibsen's reported unwillingness ever to expose himself, even during a medical examination, suggests a fear of sexuality.

The English psychiatrist, Anthony Storr, in a letter to Michael Meyer suggested that Ibsen fitted the description 'obsessional character' and wrote: 'Creative people of this temperament may be led into creativity because they (a) want to create an imaginary world in which everything can be controlled, and (b) want to avoid the unpredictability and spontaneity of real relationships with real people.'

Howard Hughes (1905–1976)

Howard Hughes was a playboy, film producer and aircraft manufacturer. Handsome, dashing and daring were adjectives used to describe Hughes as a young man. He collected properties, aircraft and glamorous women with ruthless determination. If we are to believe the stories, Hughes was devious, Machiavellian in business dealing and employed the most suspect of methods for hunting females. However, despite his distance from the kind of 'philosophical obsessionality' with which we have been primarily concerned so far in this chapter, Hughes is a classic case of obsessional illness. The public image of Hughes as a devious eccentric conveys only one aspect of the truth; it is less widely known that he made a major contribution to the development of aeronautics.

Childhood

Howard Robard Hughes was born on 24 December 1905 in Houston, Texas, the birth being a difficult one. His father had founded a successful business that made oil-drilling equipment. Hughes' mother, Allene, suffered from an intense cat-phobia (his grandmother was also strongly phobic). The young Howard was described as polite, shy, quiet and withdrawn but also characterised by a determination to succeed at the tasks he undertook. He was fascinated by mechanical gadgets, inventing a novel form of motorcycle when he was 14 years of age.

In their excellent biography, Donald Barlett and James Steele described how his mother 'smothered Howard Jr with care'. His physical condition was constantly monitored for the slightest sign of trouble and he was made to take mineral oil each night. They observed:

> 'During Howard's childhood, Allene Hughes exerted an overpowering influence on his development. She was obsessed with her son's physical and emotional condition. If she was not worried about his digestion, feet, teeth, bowels, colour, cheeks, weight, or proximity to others with contagious diseases, she was anxious about what she called his "supersensitiveness", nervousness, and inability to make friends with other boys. If Howard had no inherent anxieties in those directions as a small boy, he certainly had them by the time he reached adolescence. His mother helped instil in him lifelong phobias about his physical and mental state. Howard also learned from her that the best way to attract

attention or to escape unpleasant situations was to complain of illness. The slightest whimper from him would unleash a wave of smothering attention from Allene Hughes, and throughout his life he would pretend to be sick when he wanted to avoid responsibility or elicit sympathy.'

Howard was sent to an exclusive school in West Newton, Massachusetts. The records of his days there describe a shy and withdrawn boy, not much involved in the social life. However, he still tended to stand out on account of his height and good looks. Later he was enrolled at school in Ojai, California, where he again tended to avoid group activities, spending hours riding alone in the hills. While at Ojai, Howard learned of the death of his mother at the age of 39. He gave no open display of grief, but it might be significant that thereafter when in Houston he avoided the family home. Less than two years later, he suffered the loss of his father. His biographers believe that these two premature losses had a profound effect on consolidating Howard's own well-instilled fears for his own health. From this time onwards he was thrown into a panic by any mild irregularity in his physical condition. With the help of pills and other means, he started to protect himself from the dangers of the world.

Adult life

At first, in spite of wealth and good looks, Hughes' social incompetence rendered him something of a flop with girls. He did manage to get married but the marriage was not a success; Hughes was too much of a workaholic to allow the necessary social life and sharing. He was able to combine his two great loves – films and aircraft – by producing movies about planes, in which he did some of the flying. Sometimes he would work for stretches of up to 36 hours and earned a reputation for extreme ambition and determination. In filming, he set perfectionist and 'impossible' goals, but managed to meet them.

In spite of a lack of social skills, fame brought with it the reward of a succession of glamorous women. However, he remained self-conscious and reticent, looking distinctly ill at ease at social gatherings. The contrast between the dashing, fearless test-pilot and the shy, 'highly strung', self-effacing image that the public saw created an air of mystery around him.

In business life, Hughes earned a reputation for interfering, an inability to delegate. He demanded total control over all of his empire.

Yet Hughes was unable to make decisions himself, engaging in lengthy and disastrous procrastination, unable to distinguish the trivial from the profound. Perfectionist traits were evident even in relatively insignificant aspects of his work. His instructions were meticulous: for instance, visitors were even told in exact detail how they should park their cars and walk towards where Howard would meet them. In technical matters concerned with aircraft production, Hughes had an astonishing, almost photographic, memory. Essentially a self-taught man, with very little formal education in aeronautical science, Hughes impressed a number of the country's foremost engineers with his understanding. His round-the-world flights were planned with the obsessional's capacity for thoroughness.

Even by Hollywood's liberal standards, Hughes was a distinct eccentric, a maverick, a loner who had a taste for the sensational and a love of being seen to be doing weird and wonderful things. In 1944, Hughes suffered his first mental breakdown.

In 1946 he was injured in a crash while on a test flight. To overcome the pain, he was given morphine, and then, as a substitute, codeine. He developed a life-long addiction to codeine. Now Hughes' behaviour, always eccentric, was becoming bizarre in the extreme. Paranoia dictated that business meetings should be held either in cars parked in remote back streets or in a bathroom with the tap turned on to mask the conversation. People were now seen as germ carriers, and elaborate schemes were put into place to protect Hughes.

Insight into obsessionality

Becoming a recluse, Hughes' whole lifestyle was dictated by his obsession with hidden germs. Curtains were permanently closed, and windows and doors were sealed with masking tape. Everything became a potential menace; even the glance of a friend came to threaten contamination. Meticulous specifications were given to aides on how to protect him from germs; no threat seemed too bizarre to be considered. Earlier food fads were now accentuated, meals being taken only in the form of elaborate rituals. Another aspect of his obsession involved the abhorrence that part of his body might be wasted; hence Hughes' insistence that his urine should not be flushed down the toilet but stored in bottles instead. His fear that his perspiration would be wasted prevented him from taking baths.

One of his aides, Bob Roberts, described 'The Old Man' sitting in a chair staring at the wall. The room was insulated to prevent germs entering in the air. Hughes was naked except for a napkin spread over his groin. He resembled an emaciated skeleton, like a survivor from a concentration camp. His hair was white and dirty, and it reached the middle of his back. The toenails and fingernails were some six inches in length. Hughes' doctor was allowed neither to touch him nor speak to him, having to communicate by writing notes on a pad. In the meantime, Hughes would himself struggle to cope with his haemorrhoids, using his fingers with their six-inch nails.

Donald Barlett and James Steele wrote: 'If Howard Hughes had had a friend in the world in 1958, that person would now have encouraged or arranged psychiatric care for him before it was too late.' In contrast, the highly paid aides who surrounded Hughes did everything to cater for his every eccentric wish. This strengthened, rather than undermined, his conviction that both he and his second wife were under permanent threat from hidden germs. Also, by taking massive quantities of codeine by intravenous injection and Valium (28 times the recommended daily dose) orally, Hughes was poisoning his body. For the last 15 or so years of his life, Hughes never left his bedroom. Indeed, he hardly left his bed except to make visits to the toilet. Interminable hours were spent watching TV movies, while lying naked on dirty sheets and surrounded by piles of magazines.

Hughes died a 93-pound 'skeleton'. He had never been able to enjoy the friendship of anyone and spent most of his married state living apart from his two wives. But in a sense he died as he lived – an enigma, an eccentric, always in the gaze of publicity, an object of (now morbid) curiosity. As Donald Barlett and James Steele expressed it, 'His shyness notwithstanding, the public spotlight was his oldest addiction.'

Hughes serves to illustrate that there is a grey area between obsessions and phobias. He could probably be described equally well as having a germ phobia or an obsession about germs. Two possible extreme strategies are sometimes followed by someone with a fear of germs: extensive washing rituals or withdrawal from possible contamination. These might be termed *active* and *passive* coping strategies, respectively. Hughes adopted a predominantly passive strategy. There are records of other people who, having fears similar to Hughes', also switched from an active to a passive strategy. The irony is that either strategy taken to extremes actually brings the victims nearer to the feared object. Hands made raw by washing in detergent can be particularly vulnerable to infection. Similarly, by lying in filth, afraid to interact with an apparently hostile world, Hughes greatly increased his chances of infection with the hepatitis that he so dreaded.

Kurt Gödel (1906–1978)

The mathematician, logician and philosopher Kurt Gödel was a pioneering thinker who provided some of the 20th century's foundations to mathematics and computer science. Gödel had a very rich imagination and was able to envisage universes where time-travel into the past is possible, and he presented philosophical arguments for the existence of God. The term 'incompleteness theorem' is associated with Gödel, who also worked on relativity theory. Gödel's intellectual quest was to find rationality in all things. It is a pity that his own life suffered from a failure to extend such a principle to himself.

During the oral examination for gaining his doctorate, S Kochen remembers that he was asked to name five theorems of Gödel. The point of this question was that each and every one of those five theorems was the beginning of a whole branch of modern mathematical logic. Mathematical logic now has an established place in mathematics due to pioneers such as Gödel, Turing and others. Gödel taught few courses, did not have direct students and followers, and did not publish much, but his influence on contemporary logic, computer sciences and philosophy is immense. He foresaw the important role computers would play in the future. Gödel's theorems are at the core of contemporary discussions on the similarities and differences between human and artificial (computer) intelligence.

Roots of obsessionality

Rudolf Gödel remembered that, at about the age of eight, his brother Kurt contracted rheumatic fever, a possible complication of which could be damage to his heart. Kurt did not have any obvious physical problems after the disease but, having learned about the possibility of a cardiac effect, convinced himself that his heart was affected. Rudolf believed that this was the start of Kurt's life-long hypochondria. It probably started an obsessional attitude to his health and diet, which dominated Kurt's life ever after. Such problems resulted in his keeping daily records of body temperature and bowel functioning. This obsession developed into a fear of poisoning, either accidental or deliberate. Gödel's girlfriend and, later, wife, Adele Porkert, served as a taster and protector, helping to reduce his fears that someone was trying to poison him. Another manifestation of Gödel's obsessional fears was gas poisoning. These gases might come from the heating system or the refrigerator. He read extensively about toxicology and intoxication, especially about carbon monoxide poisoning. However, a fear of gas poisoning could have some rational basis: all the Viennese apartments in which Gödel lived at that time were heated with coal. This points to cultural factors that can influence obsessional thinking; obsessions can build on such fears.

Moving to the USA

The fear of poisonous gases had a serious repercussion when Gödel later settled in the USA. A year after his arrival at Princeton in 1940, Gödel's colleagues were seriously alarmed and contacted his physician. They wrote: 'the evidence we have had here of Dr Gödel's difficulties comes from the fact that he thinks the radiators and icebox in his apartment give off some kind of poison gas. He has accordingly had them removed, which makes the apartment a pretty uncomfortable place in the winter time.' Later '[Gödel] seems to have no such distrust of the heating plants at the Institute and . . . carries on his work here very successfully.' Gödel's immediate colleagues were assured by his doctor that his psychological problems were unlikely to take a violent form. However, based on a fear of his mental state, the institute in which Gödel worked was reluctant – until 1946 – to grant him a permanent position.

In recollections about Gödel, a neighbour, George Brown (a research associate in Princeton), described another obsessional fear: during the war years Kurt did not like to leave his apartment because of his fear that foreign visitors to town might try to kill him. Indeed, according to Brown, Kurt did not want to meet even with well-known mathematicians (one of whom was the topologist Eduard Czech). Albert Einstein and then the economist Oskar Morgenstern helped to look after Gödel, taking long walks as part of the routine that kept him functioning.

Gödel's pedantic/obsessional nature influenced many aspects of his life. In 1947, during his citizenship hearings, he expected to be questioned on the American Constitution and system of government. Gödel prepared thoroughly for the examination. Indeed, he found some inconsistency in the Constitution, which he immediately reported to

Morgenstern and Einstein. Both were amused and worried, thinking that this could create a serious problem at the hearing.

When the day of the hearing arrived, Einstein distracted Gödel with rather sombre jokes, such as 'This is next-to-last test, the last being when you step into your grave', or comparing autograph hunters with 'spirit cannibals'. On their arrival at the court, the judge invited all three of them into the chamber and, after talking for some time to Einstein, turned to Gödel and asked whether in a country such as America a dictatorship similar to Germany's would be possible. At this point Gödel, ever with an obsessional's eye for detail and incongruity, gave a positive answer followed by a broad and lengthy explanation as to how and why it is possible, quoting the feature of the Constitution that might permit this to happen.

Decline

During the last decade of his life, Gödel's decline was tragic. He convinced himself that he suffered from a heart problem, which was psychosomatic rather than physical. His concern with nutrition, body temperature and bowel habits got worse and manifested in even more excessive medication and laxatives. According to Morgenstern, by 1974 Gödel was taking a large range of different medicines for digestive, bowel and cardiac problems and for kidney and bladder infections. It is amazing that Gödel was able to survive despite taking all these medications.

When in 1977 Adele was hospitalised for six months, no one was around to taste his food. Hence, Gödel's fears of poisoning resulted in self-starvation and subsequently in death. The death certificate reads that Gödel died from 'malnutrition and inanition' (he weighed only 65 pounds) resulting from 'personality disturbance'.

For Adele Gödel, the death of her husband was an overwhelming tragedy. She struggled for him for nearly 50 years: she was his food tester, nurse, defender and protector from his many fears. Without her tolerance, persuasion, persistence and love in dealing with his psychological problems and physical needs, Gödel might never have achieved what he did. Adele Gödel – not understanding what exactly her husband did and meant for science but firmly believing in his greatness – was the stabilising factor of Kurt Gödel's life.

Essence of beliefs and reflection on a life

Four main convictions and beliefs were essential in Gödel's life:

- The universe is organised rationally and is understandable to the human mind.

- The universe is 'causally deterministic' (i.e. it can be understood in terms of one event causing another).

- There is a dualism of mind and body (i.e. the mind is something with an existence distinct from the physical body).

- Introspection (looking in at one's own mind) lies at the root of human knowledge and conceptual understanding.

One might speculate that the last of these – introspection – could, when taken to extremes, be a factor behind Gödel's hypochondria, obsessions and paranoia.

Psychologists know that in OCD ideas are logically constructed and systematised, and seem to be very convincing to the sufferer. One might suggest that the fact that Gödel was, and still is, the world's leading logician made him even more susceptible to the condition.

Comparison between Darwin and Gödel

It is interesting to compare the two great scientists Darwin and Gödel. Both made outstanding discoveries, which exceeded their own scientific expectations and put them in the spotlight. In each case, these discoveries came after extensive thought, and they changed the way that scientists view the world. Both persisted in their investigations in spite of the psychological problems that influenced their lives. Neither of them was very sociable. They lived quietly with their devoted wives and a small group of friends. By today's standards, both published rather little but were able very convincingly to pay particular ('obsessive') attention to detail.

However, some differences are also worth highlighting. Darwin's theory of evolution triggered huge opposition, driven in part by theological considerations. The theory of evolution has filtered down to a lay level of understanding, as expressed in such popular terms as 'survival of the fittest'. By contrast, Gödel's insights were not widely disseminated. Indeed, only in the last decade of the 20th century did his theorems reach anything even vaguely resembling the 'popular imagination', in the context of the discussion on human versus artificial intelligence. Whereas Darwin's scientific observations and achievements transformed him from a person with a religious faith into an agnostic, Gödel remained all his life a firm believer trying to justify and explain creation.

Glenn Gould (1932–1982)

Born in 1932, in Toronto, Glenn Gould was an only child and appeared 'rather late' (Glenn's mother was in her forties when he was born). Glenn started learning the piano at the age of three and by five was already composing. When 14, he graduated from the Toronto Conservatory, the youngest graduate ever. In 1955, he made his US debut at New York's Town Hall; it was a success, and the next day Columbia signed a recording contract with him. This sensational event catapulted Glenn Gould into world fame, the power of recording leading to a marathon of concerts. He was the first North American to play in the Soviet Union during the Cold War. Gould was the centre of attention everywhere he went or performed. However, deep down he felt very unhappy and dreaded live performances. So, in 1964 in Chicago, at the age of 32, he gave his last live performance. His career as a concert pianist was over.

Childhood and psychology

According to the recollections by Gould's father, from infancy Glenn was a 'different' child and 'liked to sing already at birth'. The parents, themselves passionate about music, were delighted, perceived the musical talent of their newborn and supported this in every way.

One might have thought that some 'differences' should have been alarming for the parents, but they were not; their reaction was one of amusement rather than apprehension. His father remembers that, even as a child, Glenn had developed a serious anxiety about his fingers.

'From the time he was a tiny child, if you rolled a ball across the floor, he'd turn and get upset and wouldn't let it touch his hands at all. He always had that sensitivity to balls. He wouldn't have anything to do with them at all, wouldn't touch the ball. It was a natural way of protecting his hands, I think. It was just the instinct not to hurt his fingers.'

Even as a schoolboy, he – being totally petrified – refused to touch a ball. At the age of four, Glenn developed an over-sensitivity to strong, bright colours. Later in life in an interview he said: 'I hate clear days; I hate sunlight; I hate yellow. Grey for me, the ultimate that one could achieve in the world.'

Glenn's mother exhibited paranoia in her concern for his health. She was constantly worried about his complexion and did not allow Glenn to be near anyone with the slightest hint of sickness. When he was a child, she warned Glenn not to go to any events where there were many people. He was not to approach crowds, in order to avoid germs and contamination. It is perhaps not surprising that Glenn developed a fear of germs and crowds, and was terrified of becoming ill.

When Glenn's mother had a stroke, he was very concerned about her condition but never visited her in hospital. The fear of getting ill and contamination from the hospital was very strong. However, Glenn did talk to her over the telephone for many hours before she lost consciousness. The death of his mother was a devastating and traumatic event, which left a deep scar on Glenn's life and made him even more introspective. She was one of the most important figures in his life – the only woman who understood his personality, who firmly believed in his musical genius and with whom he could share the successes and disappointments in his career and exchange ideas.

While at school, Glenn saw another boy become physically ill in public and noticed how everyone looked at the poor child. This episode, according to his recollection, started his fear of being ill in public, of being looked at and the fear of humiliation. After this, Glenn returned to school with a couple of mints in his pocket, which were soon supplemented by aspirin and then by more pills. Every day, he counted the seconds remaining to the end of the lessons and prayed that nothing would humiliate him.

Professional life and psychological disorder

Anxiety about his fingers together with the fear of crowds led to a rather fundamental problem with audiences. According to Gould himself, he did not like performing in public because of the horrible feeling that three thousand pairs of eyes were watching what he was doing rather than listening. Glenn developed several strategies to deal with stage-fright. One was to pretend that there was no audience, another was to convince himself that he had power over the people present.

The most reliable, however, was the strategy that had already developed into a habit: taking sedatives before going on stage. This was Glenn's way of self-control.

All these fears manifested themselves in rather 'eccentric' behaviour: overdressing – coat, hat, scarf and gloves, even in the middle of summer. He was hypersensitive to bodily functions and sensation – anything could be the symptom of disease. Gould felt that most of his fears were of psychosomatic origin. Before concerts in Russia, Gould had an attack of an eating disorder triggered by psychological factors. He was terrified by the prospect of the Russian trip, imagining that he would vomit at an important embassy dinner and that the press would love his humiliation. Glenn confessed that the fears got worse over the years. What was once just fear of eating in public developed into a fear of people and even of the thought of eating.

However, at that time – 1955 – the idea of seeking professional help for such a problem carried the stigma of being 'crazy'. Although everyone talked about his eccentric behaviour, Gould and his managers didn't want him to acquire the reputation of being mad. Nevertheless, Glenn saw a number of doctors through his life, but the treatment was always Glenn's own affair and he and only he made decisions about the medication he took. Usually the medication was a combination of all the prescriptions from different doctors and his own efforts at self-medication.

His friends were very concerned about Gould's drug taking and the ease with which he took them. He would pop a couple of Valium as a matter of course, or when he feared confrontations. In addition, he would take an all-purpose drug cocktail consisting of barbiturates and caffeine among other things for headaches, as well as antibiotics for infections and various tranquillisers for emotion disorders.

Less than a year after his mother died, Glenn was diagnosed with high blood pressure (hypertension). He immediately started taking detailed records of his blood pressure. Then, fearing that the American-made apparatus for measuring blood pressure was not correct, he bought another two – Japanese and German – to compare the readings. April 24, for example, contained eleven entries, with an interval between 5.30 a.m. and 2.30 p.m. when Glenn usually slept. His pulse rate was another worry, and the pulse chart for 18 January 1977 has 20 entries with details such as 'phone conversation' or 'WC' among others.

After 1967, Gould stopped flying because of his fear of being killed in a crash. This seems to have been influenced by the fact that some famous musicians (William Kapell, Jacques Thibaud) had been killed in an aeroplane crash. To reach the various concert venues, he now relied on trains and cars.

Gould had a number of ritualistic behaviours. For example, he would perform only if he could use his own chair, which he carried everywhere with him. He would hold his hands and arms in very hot water before each performance or recording session. Various fears contributed to Gould's decision to retire from the stage. He gave his last recital on 28 March 1964, when he was only 32 years old. The performing career of the highest paid Canadian was over. But the ritualistic behaviour remained. Moreover, some rituals were added: a piano technician should be on stand-by duty when he was recording, and any recording sessions must be done at night.

Perfectionism and control

Something else contributed to his retirement: an obsessional trait of perfectionism. As Glenn himself put it, one cannot have a 'take two' in front of a live audience. While making his first studio recording, Gould discovered the magic of technology. He was able to repeat and correct his performance until the musical sound was *perfect*. The record producer can create a disc made up of the best parts of numerous 'takes', whereas at a concert it is always 'take 1' whether good or bad. Gould called this 'non-take-twoness'.

In an interview, Yehudi Menuhin explained that Gould 'did not like a situation where he was not in *total control* – of music, of the people, of the voices'.

The enigma

Usually the sales of records go down if the artist is not performing live but this did not happen in Gould's case. A whole new generation of fans appeared without hearing their legend in public. Through his seclusion and clever manipulation of the media, everything Gould wanted to be known was recorded, written and broadcast. He created a living legend about himself – an eccentric, clever, sharp person, who either did not have a personal life or whose personal life was very unremarkable. Glenn Gould became even more famous and he remains a best-seller. Gould wanted to be left alone, to be in control of his performance and his life.

Gould needed people and human contact as well, but the terms and conditions of these contacts should be his. He spent an enormous amount of time talking, usually in the middle of the night. These long-distance telephone conversations were made without any concern for the other person's need for sleep, and the issues discussed were those he was comfortable with. If somebody tried to contact Glenn, the answering machine was always there but he would rarely return the call and only when *he* was ready.

Superstition

Towards the end of his life superstitions about death became evident and he was concerned that no one would come to his funeral. He was led to ruminate about the superstition held by the composer Schönberg that his age of death would be divisible by 13. Apparently, Schönberg passed 65 and might have been expected to have been able to look forward to at least the years until the age of 78. However, Gould was then struck by the superstition that it is a bad omen not only if the number is divisible by 13 but also if the two digits of the year add up to 13. In fact, he passed his 49th year but died at the young age of 50. Glenn's final fears were unwarranted: crowds attended his funeral.

Woody Allen (1935–)

Perhaps the best-known and best-loved obsessional is Woody Allen, who manages to weave into his jokes and screen characters themes from his own ruminations and fear of death. This is brilliantly illustrated in such films as *Love and Death* and *Hannah and her Sisters*. In interviews, Allen has conveyed his anxiety:

'The fundamental thing behind all motivation and all activity is the constant struggle against annihilation and against death. It's absolutely stupefying in its terror, and it renders anyone's accomplishments meaningless.'

Allen expresses a terror at the prospect that the universe might one day not exist. What is the point of struggling for artistic perfection in the midst of such a precarious existence? Yet the same creative talent can give us:

'I do not believe in an afterlife, although I am bringing a change of underwear.'

and

> 'It's not that I'm afraid to die. I just don't want to be there when it happens.'

Studying Allen is not always easy. Though he undoubtedly incorporates features of his worst fears into his films, these works should not simply be taken as autobiographical. He shows a certain suspicion of interviews, books and articles that describe his life. However, there is sufficient reliable information, some of it written by Allen himself, to give a fairly clear picture. Several well-written biographies exist and they reveal an impressive consensus of opinion.

Childhood

He was born Alan Stewart Konigsberg on 1 December 1935 at Flatbush, a middle-class and then predominantly Jewish district in Brooklyn, New York City. Woody seems to have been reclusive as a child, spending most of his time hidden away in his room pursuing, among other things, magic. There seem to have been rather few friends. He didn't fit well into the school system and made little impression on his teachers, being essentially self-involved. On his own, Woody showed enormous persistence at tasks he chose to be interested in, particularly perfecting his music and conjuring tricks. There is some evidence that he was bullied by bigger boys at times; his small build, shortness and red hair might have contributed. He seems to have had little or no success regarding girlfriends. However, even at school, he had an unusual talent for writing gags and jokes, for which he was able to earn a considerable amount.

Adult life

Allen dropped out of college and survived somewhat precariously as a writer of humorous material for comedians, a very different career from that of doctor or lawyer, which a respectable Jewish mother would have wished for her son. Allen read a lot; Samuel Johnson, James Boswell, Sigmund Freud and Søren Kierkegaard were among his favourite writers. Fundamental issues of life, death and God, as depicted in the work of Kafka, Dostoevsky and the film director Ingmar Bergman, held his fascination. By stages Allen was to develop into a film actor, writer and director, and to acquire the image known to millions, neurotic on screen as well as off, under psychoanalysis, inordinately fascinated by death, God and sex, chronically shy and prone to fads, and being anhedonic – tending to turn pleasure into sorrow. (The film title *Annie Hall* derives from the original intended title *Anhedonia*.)

Insights into obsessionality

Aspects of Allen's life reveal the obsessional's love of creating predictability and control, to be a creature of habit. For example, it is widely reported that, while filming *What's New Pussycat?* in Paris, he ate the same meal for six months – soup of the day and sole. By all accounts Allen is extremely well disciplined and controlled. In addition, the real image is one characterised by scrupulous honesty, moral integrity and traits of extreme 'workaholism' and perfectionism. A 15-hour writing day is not uncommon.

Lee Guthrie's *Woody Allen: a biography* reveals another aspect of Allen's make-up – that he tends to wish he were doing something other than what he is doing. This is a bizarre kind of extreme optimism shared with other obsessionals. 'I always think the next thing I do will be fun. Then when I do it I don't like it at all.' Guthrie also quoted Allen as describing himself as egotistical and vain.

Writing in *Time* magazine, film critic Richard Schickel observed:

'The basic Woody persona has always been a well-loved figure, a projection of the modern urban Everyman's privately held fantasies and terrors.'

Allen is an (if not the) undisputed genius of American cinema, combining qualities of, on the one hand, Groucho Marx and Charlie Chaplin with, on the other, Samuel Johnson and Søren Kierkegaard. A more improbable blend of talents is difficult to imagine but it works, as millions of devoted followers testify. Vincent Canby, a long-standing Woody fan and film critic of the *New York Times*, said of his hero:

'There's nobody else in American films who comes anywhere near him in originality and interest. One has to go back to Chaplin and Buster Keaton, people who were totally responsible for their own movies, to find anyone comparable.'

In her excellent biography . . . *but we need the eggs – The Magic of Woody Allen*, Diane Jacobs has made the particularly apposite observation:

'. . . the obsessions that were with him in the nightclub acts are still with him today. These obsessions have mostly to do with the incongruity of things. Why can't the body perform what the mind can conceive – such as immortality? Why can't experience imitate the perfection of art? Why is the ideal always so much finer than the practice?'

In his peculiar ability for taking the utterly familiar, spotting its latent absurdity, its inherent incongruity, and being able to express this in a brilliant wit, Allen strongly reminds us of Samuel Johnson. There is something very Johnsonian in the style of expressing private fears in stories. In his rumination over moral dilemmas, such as the ethics of whether to kill Napoleon in the film *Love and Death*, Allen displays something of the talent of Kierkegaard.

In *The Times* (12 July 1986) Caryn James noted that:

'Few artists of his stature admit to so many self doubts while displaying so much confidence; rarely is such an overwhelming need for control manifested in such a mild manner.'

James added that:

'. . . his obsession with death is so strong it must be deflected through the skewed vision of comedy. In film, he has found his perfect vehicle.'

Indeed, Allen was quoted in *Time* magazine as having said that 'death is the big obsession behind all the things I've done.' Allen has always held such a fear:

'I was always obsessed with death, even as a child. It always used to frighten me. I have memories of being very young, probably six or eight, and being put to sleep at night and lying in the black, thinking "someday I will be dead", and really focusing vivid feelings on it, a vivid attempt to imagine the emptiness, the finality, the irrevocability of it.'

Although Allen's obsession is unwanted, it is not perceived as being at all illogical or senseless. On the contrary, Eric Lax in his biography *Woody Allen and his Comedy* noted that Allen will quote Tolstoy on the subject of death: 'any man over thirty-five with whom death is not the main consideration is a fool'.

Brian Wilson (1942–)

The driving force behind one of the most successful pop-groups in history – The Beach Boys – was a fragile genius named Brian Wilson. He created the group, he wrote its music and lyrics, produced albums and made innovations to compete with leading groups such as the Beatles. Furthermore, he made the members of the group, who were his brothers and cousins, multi-millionaires. In six years, between 1962 and 1968, Brian Wilson produced 14 albums, more than 120 songs! By the time he was 23 (!) he had already written and produced his tenth album – the famous *Pet Sounds*.

Brian's history is extremely complex and involved considerable drug taking. It is not easily classified. Thus, although his life might not be considered an example of mainstream obsessionality, he seems to have certain features of this personality and disorder.

Childhood

Brian was born in 1942 to a pianist mother and songwriter father. His father – Murry Wilson – came from a very abusive family. As a child and a teenager, Murry was severely beaten by his father. On one occasion, Murry's father beat him with a lead pipe until blood splattered and a piece of his ear was cut off. The abuse carried on through generations, involving Murry's own children: he was bad tempered and often was very violent towards his wife and children. As a result of beatings by Murry, Brian became deaf in one ear.

Murry had a glass eye and, as a last resort to scare his children and exert control over them, he would take it out in front of them and put it in a glass of water. The net result was that Brian would not drink from a glass, only from a bottle. Thus, the first of Brian's fears appeared – violence and dominance by his father and the glass eye. Murry, an unsuccessful songwriter, was very jealous of Brian's ability to write music, and he never praised his son. The criticism was endless, nothing was good enough for Murry and, as a result, nothing was perfect for Brian (he was always putting himself down).

Youth

Perhaps the family atmosphere and the puzzles of human nature led Brian to think, while he was a student of El Camino Junior College, of becoming a psychologist. His reason for this was that people 'confused' him and he wanted to understand them better.

From his teens, Brian had an urge to write music. If he was not able to write, he felt physically ill. He could not sleep, he was haunted with worries and anxieties and overwhelmed by fears that he would never be able to write again. These were Brian's everyday feelings but, when on tour and needing to perform rather than write, the fears got worse. He had to write to keep the demons quiet; this was, as he himself put it, a compulsion.

The group

Brian's high standards for himself and for others gained him a reputation of being a tyrant. He pushed everyone to the limit, including in recording sessions, which lasted nine and ten hours. Brian was also a perfectionist, but the price was high. He had difficulty sleeping at night, and when he succeeded his world was full of nightmares. His mind was permanently occupied by the same word – 'better'.

By the time Brian was 22, the pressure of performing, recording and writing music was so great that he started losing control over his behaviour. He would lose the thread of conversation, easily became upset and cried, and people scared him. He was obsessed about details in music and in everyday life – for example, he would endlessly count floor tiles, or some details on the ceiling, or peas or other bits of food on a plate.

In his apartment, he could lie on the floor, or pace, or stare at objects. Brian was crying for help, but family and friends did not take his behaviour seriously, thinking that these were just his eccentricities. In order to escape and to relieve the stress, he started drinking . . . a lot. At the beginning it worked, but later, permanently intoxicated, Brian was able neither to perform nor to function properly.

Quitting

The 22-year-old Brian Wilson needed rest and psychological help. In the previous two years he had written music and lyrics, arranged and produced, played and sung in eight albums. He was driven to the edge. Alcohol was no longer an escape from obsessions and fears, so Brian came up with an idea to quit touring and performing altogether. He suddenly found a means to manipulate people. He used his oddity and announced that he was not going to perform any more. The group's reaction was, at first, disbelief; he was not taken seriously, as usual. Then came the reaction of anger and, finally, acceptance.

However, quitting performing and devoting all his time to writing music did not free Brian. He had the same problem of trying to prove to his dad and himself that he was not a loser. The fears and anxiety remained. He dreaded getting up in the morning, being anxious about the possibility of bad things happening. Thus came drugs, at first as a possible escape and 'medication', and then as a serious problem.

The long-dreaded Murry died in 1973; soon after this Brian decided to stop writing music and stay in bed. He did exactly this for more than two and a half years. After a long battle with drug abuse, undergoing unsuccessful and successful therapy and nearly breaking with the family, Brian managed to write music again and, in 1990, published an autobiography – *Wouldn't it be Nice: my own story*. He dedicated the book to his doctor, who had helped him through by suggesting small goals to be achieved one at a time and helping Brian to meet them.

Karen Carpenter (1950–1983)

Karen Carpenter must surely be one of the most tragic figures in American popular music history. Her death at the age of 32 from heart failure associated with anorexia nervosa was a shock to anyone who knew her or loved her music. Although this eating disorder has some special features that are not shared by such 'mainstream' obsessional disorders as checking and washing (e.g. the details of the kind of therapy that is appropriate), it none the less has certain features in common with these forms of OCD. In addition, it is often associated with a perfectionist personality type, as in the case of Karen Carpenter.

Karen Carpenter's life might also serve as a reminder of something that is equally applicable to Howard Hughes (see earlier in this chapter): wealth and fame do not necessarily bring the best and most prompt help. Indeed, some would even argue that, on the contrary, the rich and famous are able to exert more control over their choices and thereby pursue idiosyncratic courses of action in defiance of their own best interests.

Background

Karen Carpenter was born in 1950, the second child of music-loving parents. In contrast to her introverted brother Richard, she was an outgoing, active child. In her early teens she had a 'sweet tooth', was overweight and started hating her figure, especially her 'wide hips'. The fact that the family moved from Connecticut to California when Karen was 13 did not help. She missed her friends desperately and as a result took refuge in food.

At about this time she started playing drums and singing. Richard was the musical driving force behind their band and soon the reputation of this talented musical student of California State University and his 16-year-old sister went beyond the university campus. That everything must be perfect meant hours and hours of rehearsing. For Karen, however, the elusive quest for perfection did not end with music. The thought that her body was not perfect tormented her. She was singing, playing drums, partly managing the group and constantly worrying about her weight. She ritualistically and repeatedly weighed herself.

Becoming an adult

When Karen's first boyfriend appeared in 1966, the anxiety about her appearance led to a period of a dieting, consisting of taking water and nothing else. Alas, nobody took her dieting seriously enough. As an example of an all-too-common paradox, Karen's concern about her body being overweight grew in proportion to her loss of weight. One could speculate that in terms of eating and weight here was at least one aspect of her life over which she could gain total control.

It seems that, early on, Karen created an image of the 'perfect man' for her but alas he was not to be found. Being on the road all the time meant there was no time for relationships outside the band, so her private life did not extend beyond the Carpenters' entourage. Karen's reputation of being in control and controlling, an inflexible singer and sister was well known within the entourage, which by 1970 was around 30 people. She developed a reputation for punctuality and being pernickety about timetables and schedules. The reputation also extended to an obsession about money and jealousy of any female daring to come near to her brother.

Serious disorder

Soon after Richard and Karen moved from the family house in California, friends and family started noticing Karen's unusual eating pattern and the slim state of her body. However, everyone still thought that such a weight is healthy. She cut out eating sweets, although she had enjoyed this from childhood. The fact that by this time she was leaving almost all her food on the plate, barely touching it, should have been alarming, but it was not.

At 25 years of age this outstandingly successful woman did not see herself as such. As her biographer, Ray Coleman notes in his book *The Carpenters: the untold story*:

> 'Karen felt that to be a modern young woman, it was a requirement to be slim and beautiful, talented and assertive, intelligent and independent. In her opinion, she held only the last four cards.'

Karen was never satisfied with recordings, concerts or her personal appearance. It did not matter that fans adored her singing or that men found her attractive; she just could not see the reality and felt more and more inadequate. By now her part of the house was full of the Disney soft toys that she had been collecting since childhood (another escape from reality) and her weight was dangerously low.

The obsession of reducing her weight was growing, although she was down to 6 stone (40 kg) and too exhausted to do the scheduled European tour. Karen was hospitalised and then released on condition that she would rest and eat sensibly. She found it impossible to rest and, although very weak and exhausted, went back to an overloaded work routine.

Karen was 26 years old when she decided to move from the house that she shared with Richard. This was an independence that she craved. Unfortunately, it did not stop her feelings of inadequacy and allowed her to continue her starving habit. Visitors to Karen's apartment recalled that the kitchen was spotless, with no signs of use, and that an enormously large space was filled with toys. In the wardrobe, her clothes were arranged in immaculate order.

By now, family and friends became aware of her state and the seriousness of the problem. Her parents and Richard tried to persuade her to eat: they argued with her, screamed and even called her a bag of bones (alas, this representing a type of confrontational logic not to be recommended for any such condition whether anorexia or 'mainstream' OCD). All was in vain. The tormenting thoughts of dissatisfaction with her body and inadequacy did not go away and Karen's weight was dropping even further.

Brother and sister problems

Richard had problems of his own. Since 1971 he had been taking sleeping pills and his intake grew dangerously over the years. In 1977, he acknowledged the situation in which he found himself and underwent a detoxification programme. Thus, he began a nearly two-year battle with his addiction. It was Richard who firmly believed that Karen's eating habits should be changed. This should be not only through medication and persuasion but also by reducing the influence of obsessive thoughts and building a realistic image of herself.

In 1979, while recording a solo album, Karen was found by the producer, unconscious on the hotel floor. She admitted taking the sleeping pills that had turned Richard into an addict. However, Karen did not mention the laxatives and thyroid medication that put an additional strain on her.

The later years

Although recorded, her solo album did not appear. Karen suggested recording another album, this time with Richard. Richard set one condition: that Karen should regain some weight before any recording could start. Superficially, the threat worked and Karen gained some weight. However, deep-rooted problems remained and psychologically nothing changed.

In 1980 Karen married Tom Burris. It was a rather unexpected and a short-lived marriage (the couple separated in 1981). An extrovert lover of outdoor activities, Tom was opposite to the introverted Karen.

During 1980 Karen realised that her health needed the special attention of a doctor. She had regular sessions in New York with a Dr Levenkron, who was of the opinion that anorexia, bulimia and OCD are interrelated. According to her biographer, Ray Coleman, Dr Levenkron reported: 'Because of her surreptitious behaviour, by the time we all started intervening, we were too late. This is an alert. Here was a lovely person who didn't want to die but was unstoppable.'

After three months there was little change. Richard was convinced that Karen needed residential supervision. Karen returned to New York and checked into hospital where she was fed intravenously. She left the hospital in November 1982, weighing 7 stone (45 kg), and returned to Los Angeles.

In Los Angeles it became apparent that Karen was slipping back into her old habits. On 4 February, while staying at her parent's house, she was found collapsed in the bedroom. The cause of death was heart failure due to anorexia nervosa. Karen was not quite 33 years old.

18
Conclusion

Obsessional thoughts raise some profound questions about the nature of humans, thought and free will. To what extent do we have free will over our behaviour and pattern of thoughts? On closer examination, can we even couch this question in meaningful terms? Whatever answer is attempted to these questions needs to be qualified by the existence of people who are plagued by intrusive thoughts in spite of their attempts to get rid of them.

It would be nice to be able to draw together the various strands of this book into some clear-cut conclusions and suggestions for therapy. Unfortunately, the investigation of obsessional thoughts remains something of an enigma. To state otherwise would be to deceive you. However, we believe that some pointers are now available, hints as to what might be going on, and there is every reason to believe that such hints will prove useful leads to further investigation. Behaviour therapy and drugs that target serotonin are very effective for some people.

Brain function

Although the form of obsessionality might strike us as a puzzle, we should not be unduly surprised that behavioural systems 'go wrong'. TV sets and computers go wrong, so why not the infinitely more complex brain and behavioural systems? What is perhaps more surprising is that they normally work as well as they do. Obsessional problems probably seem all the more bizarre because the people experiencing them appear to be so 'very normal' in other respects. They seem rational, persistent and purposive in their lives. So why can't they cure themselves or be more receptive to therapy? When such a person happens to be a trained psychologist (like F.T.), the feeling that the solution should invariably lie in one's own hands must seem even stronger. But, alas, this is not always so.

Perfectionism

Caution is needed when we describe an individual as having obsessional personality traits, such as orderliness and perfectionism. Without doubt, obsessionals tend to have such traits but it should not be supposed that every aspect of their lives bears witness to meticulous planning and devotion to duty. After all, there are only 24 hours in a day and even obsessionals need to sleep. Thus extreme persistence and conscientiousness are likely to be shown in tasks that are given priority, because they serve the individual's dominant goals. Tasks at odds with these goals or that take precious time away from them might assume a much lower place in the hierarchy or even be treated with contempt. F.T. can ruminate for long periods over the use of a 'which' rather than a 'that' in a piece of writing, in the midst of chaos, unpaid bills and uncashed cheques. This aspect of obsessionality is often overlooked; perfection might well be applied in only one or two areas of life.

In other words, we would argue that any perfectionism will be apparent in the contexts of the individual's overall goals. Turning now to OCD, in the extreme, one part of the body can be the focus for washing rituals while the rest of the body remains filthy. Pierre Janet and Isaac Marks, among others, have reported visiting the homes of patients obsessed with cleanliness in, for example, the toilet, while the kitchen stinks of the rotten remains of food caked onto surfaces. One of Marks' patients, a man obsessed with cleaning away imaginary dog excrement, caught gonorrhoea from a prostitute.

Goal-directed behaviour

From both F.T.'s personal experience and an academic viewpoint, we emphasise the need to look closely at goal-direction in behaviour. Events that are in some way at odds with the dominant goals are particularly likely to cue fearful ruminations in me (F.T.). Take a case in which one might plan to fly from London to New York. You might suppose that a certain level of anticipatory fear would be associated with such an event. In my (F.T.'s) case, the frequency and level of such fears would depend upon how the visit fitted my current concerns. If the job of my dreams were waiting for me in the USA, there would be little or no fearful rumination in advance. If any were to appear, I could quickly dismiss it. If, however, I were flying half-heartedly to a New York conference that was not likely to be very valuable, the intrusions about flying might well be frequent and more intense.

Control

Another concept that emerges as being vital is that of control; obsessionals seem to have a greater need than normal to be able to exert control over their environment. This includes the physical and social environments. Thus obsessionals will seek relationships in which they can do the controlling rather than be the controlled. Interestingly, the need to exert control and *predictability* over the environment is now at the core of the study of animal welfare. The Dutch ethologist, Professor Piet Wiepkema, goes so far as to equate an absence of suffering and stress in farm animals with an ability to predict and control their environment. It would seem entirely reasonable that the obsessional human experiences a greater than normal need to possess these two capacities in a wider number of contexts. In a fascinating study entitled 'The obsessive's myth of control', Dr Allan Mallinger argues that, at one level, obsessionals can even convince themselves that they have total control over their destiny. The similarities – in terms of loss of control – between depression, stress and obsessional disorders seem worthy of further analysis.

Differences between obsessionals

We must also be careful not to see obsessionals as too much of a homogeneous group. There must be a number of common traits, of course, for the term *personality type* to have any meaning, but beyond this we should expect rich variety among obsessionals. Indeed, in some ways it is difficult to imagine a greater difference than between, say, the promiscuous and empire-building Howard Hughes and the prudish Hans Christian Andersen, or between the timid character portrayed so vividly by Woody Allen and the giant and fearless George Borrow. The weeping and forever sentimental and nostalgic Andersen, the aggressive and morose Samuel Johnson, the passionate Borrow and the anxiety-ridden Allen do not lend themselves easily to the not-uncommon textbook image of the obsessional as being emotionally flat.

F.T.'s personal views

Now for a final word on a personal level, we would like to discuss some issues arising from the book. Have I learned anything about my life from a study of the personality type that I fit and the disorder from which I have suffered? Of course, I have learned a lot and have gained inspiration from knowing that others have suffered from the same condition. I feel that it is a bit like having a wooden leg or a tendency to epilepsy – life would be much better without the difficulty or disorder but one can still make the best of it. I have lived a life rich in experiences with few fears that have actually stopped me doing things. I am not a pessimist and carrying out this study has not moved me in that direction.

My life has had 'peak experiences': at Sussex, in Odense and Copenhagen, and later while on sabbatical in France and West Germany. These were experiences that I would not have missed, escaping completely from the troubles of life. Things that have bothered me in life have done so intensely but, on the positive side, very few things have, or do, bother me. After the experience of mental breakdown, the content of so many concerns and worries of the affluent Western middle class seems to me to be of monumental triviality. This might sound arrogant but it is how I feel.

Suppose I had remained within the secure and predictable confines of my village in Cambridgeshire. Who can say what might have happened? I would have missed the stimulation of teaching Open University students, and that is an experience that I would not have missed for anything.

When times seem bad, I get much inspiration from the words of George Borrow in *Lavengro*:

> 'Reader, amidst the difficulties and dangers of this life, should you ever be tempted to despair, call to mind these latter chapters of the life of Lavengro. There are few positions, however difficult, from which dogged resolution and perseverance may not liberate you.'

Glossary

analogy a means of explanation in terms of showing that the thing to be explained is like something else that is more familiar and better understood, e.g. a computer as an analogy of the brain (similar use to 'model').

appetitive urge (or 'appetitive compulsion') an insistent urge towards *attaining* something positive such as in gambling, drug-taking or sexual contact. Distinct from OCD, where the goal is to *avoid* something.

behaviour therapy a type of therapy characterised by targeting behaviour as such and trying to alter it. In the case of OCD, this would consist of, say, exposure to the dreaded situation.

behavioural modelling a version of behaviour therapy in which the therapist engages in the activity that causes distress to the patient. The rationale is that patient will learn to imitate ('model') the therapist.

brain lock a version of behaviour therapy pioneered by Dr Jeffrey Schwartz and described in the book of that name.

checking repeatedly inspecting something such as a gas tap or door to see that it is in the desired state.

chemical messenger a chemical, for example serotonin or dopamine, that conveys signals from one of the brain's neurons (nerve cells) to another. Sometimes called 'neurotransmitter'.

cognitive restructuring the process of altering a patient's thought processes by some means. It can occur as part of cognitive therapy by exploring the implications of the thoughts.

cognitive therapy a professional technique that looks at the interpretation that is put on the obsessional thoughts and tries to modify this. It is a process of trying to get the patient to see the thoughts in a new light.

conditioning a process of learning in which a previously neutral event is given significance as a result of its pairing with something important. For example, as studied by Pavlov, an otherwise insignificant event like a tone can come to evoke salivation by pairing with food or fear by pairing with trauma.

existential dilemma a term relating to 'existence in the world' and describing the dilemma confronting an individual in coming to terms with such things as mortality.

existential terror a terror at the nature of the human condition and existence, i.e. its insecure and transient nature.

exposure technique a technique whereby a patient is deliberately exposed to the content of their obsession but without taking corrective ('compulsive') action in response to it; e.g. exposure to 'contaminated' hands or a spoken version of their obsession played over headphones.

model an aid to description and understanding. As such, something having certain features in common with the target. Used here in the sense of (1) explanatory or theoretical model, an attempt to explain something by pointing to something with which it is similar (e.g. the disease *model* of OCD points to features of OCD that are like diseases) and (2) the therapist as *model* in undertaking a task that the patient fears.

morbid preoccupation a state of repetitive intrusion into conscious awareness of unpleasant thoughts that have a logical link to events in the person's life; e.g. someone constantly occupied by thoughts of their child's welfare while the child is in hospital.

neurosis a psychological disorder in which the patient does not lose contact with conventional rationality. It includes anxiety, depression and OCD. Contrast with 'psychosis'.

neutralisation the process of finding or attempting to find a thought that counters the intrusion. What might seem to be a process of neutralisation could be serving to reinforce the obsessional intrusions.

neutralising thought a thought that follows and seems to counter the obsessional thought. However, in reality, its emergence might be a factor reinforcing the obsessional intrusion.

OCD *see* obsessive compulsive disorder

obsession a thought that is unwanted but which imposes itself upon the conscious mind.

obsessional personality a personality type that is characterised by a range of such traits as conscientiousness, reliability and perfectionism. It is often thought to predispose to OCD but there is not a necessary link between having the personality and acquiring the disorder.

obsessive compulsive disorder (OCD) also termed 'obsessio*nal* compulsive disorder'. A disorder characterised by intrusive thoughts and compulsive activity, whether in the form of behaviour or mental activity.

obsessive phobia a condition that combines features of both OCD and a phobia; e.g. a fear of dogs because of a belief that a loose dog hair could trigger a particular disorder.

paradoxical intention a technique that involves trying to exaggerate ('ridicule') the nature of the intrusive thought and trying to live with this exaggerated form. The hope is that the initial thought will thereby lose its impact.

phobia an exaggerated fear of a particular thing, such as heights or spiders.

premonition an experience in which the person feels that something bad is going to happen (compare 'obsession').

psychoanalysis/psychoanalytic a school of psychology most closely associated with Sigmund Freud. The emphasis is on the dynamics of unconscious and conscious thought processes and how to interpret their content.

psychoanalyst a practitioner of the technique of psychoanalysis.

psychosis mental disorder characterised by a lack of contact with reality; e.g. schizophrenia. In lay terms, associated with madness. Contrast with 'neurosis'.

psychotic to describe a psychosis, which see.

pure obsession a controversial term. Sometimes used to describe the experience of obsession without associated behaviour. However, some argue that this term detracts from compulsive mental activity, which will almost always accompany any obsession.

pure ruminator *see* pure obsession

reinforcer something that follows a thought or behaviour and tends to strengthen it, i.e. makes it more likely to happen in the future.

response prevention part of the technique of exposure therapy. The patient is urged in the presence of the therapist not to perform the compulsive behaviour.

ritual a sequence of actions with some end-point in mind; e.g. to produce rain. This might be part of a religious ceremony and cause no problem but it might be pathological.

rumination perhaps most usually used to describe a chewing of something in the mouth. As used here, to describe a mental 'chewing over' of ideas.

schizophrenia an example of a psychosis in which the mind is flooded with strange images that are convincing; e.g. that, in an extreme case, the sufferer is Napoleon or that little green men are hiding in the garden.

selective serotonin reuptake inhibitor a class of drug used for treating OCD (e.g. Prozac). It acts by targeting serotonin, one of the brain's chemical messengers.

serotonin one of the brain's chemical messengers (also known as a 'transmitter' or a 'neurotransmitter').

thought stopping a technique used to get rid of an unwanted thought; e.g. saying out loud or under one's breath 'Stop!' whenever the unwanted thought appears.

tic repetitive 'involuntary' action involving *only a part* of the body, such as a facial grimace or jutting out a leg.

Resources

Publications about OCD

Brain Lock by Jeffrey Schwartz (1997) London: HarperCollins

Living with Fear by Isaac Marks (1978) Maidenhead: McGraw-Hill

Obsessive Compulsive Disorders: a complete guide to getting well and staying well by Fred Penzel (1999) London: Jessica Kingsley

Obsessive Compulsive Disorder: the facts, 2nd edition by Padmal De Silva and Stanley Rachman (1998) Oxford: Oxford University Press

Obsessive Compulsive Disorders by Fred Penzel (2001) Oxford: Oxford University Press

OCD in Children and Adolescents by John S March and Karen Mulle (1998) London: Guilford Press

Understanding Obsessions and Compulsions by Frank Tallis (1992) London: Sheldon Press

Understanding Obsessive Compulsive Disorder by Fiona Hill (2000) London: Mind

American titles

The Boy who Couldn't Stop Washing by Judith L Rapoport (1997) New American Library (ISBN 0 45117202 7)

Childhood Obsessive Compulsive Disorder by G Francis (1996) Sage Publications (ISBN 0 80395922 2)

Getting Control: Overcoming Your Obsession and Compulsions by Lee Baer (2000) Plume Books (ISBN 0 45228177 6)

Obsessive Compulsive Disorder by Herbert L Gravitz and James W Broatch (1998) Partners Publishing Group (ISBN 0 96611044 7)

Obsessive-Compulsive Disorder: help for Children and Adolescents (Patients-Centered Guides) by Mitzi Waltz (2000) O'Reilly & Associates (ISBN 1 56592758 3)

Obsessive Compulsive Disorder in Children and Adolescents edited by Judith L Rapoport (1989) American Psychiatric Publishing (ISBN 0 99049292 6)

Obsessive Compulsive Disorder: a survival guide for family and friends by C Roy (1993) Obsessive Compulsive Anonymous (ISBN 0 96280661 7)

The OCD Workbook: your guide to breaking free from obsessive compulsive disorder by Bruce M Hyman and Cherry Pedrick (1999) New Harbinger Publications (ISBN 1 57224169 1)

Polly's Magic Games by C Foster (1994) Dilligaf Publications (ISBN 0 96390708 5)

When Once is Not Enough: help for obsessive compulsives by Gail Steketee and Kerrin White (1991) New Harbinger Publications (ISBN 0 93498687 8)

For a basic introduction to the principles of biological psychology

Biological Psychology: An Integrative Approach by Frederick Toates (2001) Harlow: Prentice-Hall

Leaflets

Mental Health and Growing Up A series containing 36 fact-sheets on a range of common mental health problems, including discipline, behavioural problems and conduct disorder, and stimulant medication.
To order the pack, contact:
Book Sales
Royal College of Psychiatrists
17 Belgrave Square
London SW1X 8PG
Tel: 020 7235 2351, ext. 146
Fax: 020 7245 1231
E-mail: booksales@rcpsych.ac.uk

Organisations and websites concerned with OCD

Useful organisations

Anxiety Care
Cardinal Heenan Centre
326 High Road
Ilford
Essex IG1 1QP
Tel: 020 8262 8891
Website: www.anxietycare.org.uk
A mental-health charity, it helps individuals with recovery from neurotic disorders.

First Steps to Freedom
7 Avon Court
School Lane
Kenilworth
Warwickshire CV8 2GX
Tel: 01926 864473
Fax: 0870 164 0567
Website: www.first-steps.org
A self-help group for various disorders, including OCD.

Mental Health Foundation
20/21 Cornwall Terrace
London NW1 4QL
Tel: 020 7535 7400
Fax: 020 7535 7474
Website: www.mentalhealth.org.uk
A mental health charity with an emphasis on campaigning for better insight into disorders.

MIND – The Mental Health Charity
15–19 Broadway
London E15 4BQ
Tel: 020 8519 2122
Fax: 020 8522 1725
Website: www.mind.org.uk/index.asp
A mental health charity that works both at the level of campaigning and with help to sufferers.

National Phobics Society
Zion Community Resource
   Centre
339 Stretford Road
Hulme
Manchester M15 4ZY
Tel: 0870 7700 456
Fax: 0161 227 9862
Website: www.phobics-society.org.uk
A charity specialising in help for people with phobias.

No Panic
93 Brands Farm Way
Randlay
Telford TF3 2JQ
Tel: 01952 590545
Helpline: 10 a.m.–10 p.m. daily
Website: www.no-panic.co.uk
A self-help group for people who have panic attacks, phobias and obsessive compulsive disorders. Based on self-help through local group meetings and telephone groups.

OAASIS – Office for Advice Assistance Support & Information on Special Needs
Brock House
Grigg Lane
Brockenhurst
Hampshire SO42 7RE
Helpline: 09068 633 201
Fax: 01590 622 687
Website:
www.nottssnn.freeserve.co.uk/oaasis/index.html
A charity specialising in advice for parents of children with mental health problems.

Obsessive Action
Aberdeen Centre
22–24 Highbury Grove
London N5 2EA
Helpline: 020 7226 4000
Fax: 020 7288 0828
Website:
www.obsessive-action.demon.co.uk
The main British charity for people with OCD. It provides sources of information designed to help sufferers and works to raise public understanding of OCD.

Samaritans
10 The Grove
Slough
Berkshire SL1 1QP
Tel: 01753 216 500
Fax: 01753 775 787
Website: www.samaritans.org.uk
An organisation to bring help to people in great distress from whatever cause. To talk to someone, ring 08457 90 90 90.

Sane
1st Floor, Cityside House
40 Adler Street
London E1 1EE
Tel: 020 7375 1002
Fax: 020 7375 2162
Website: www.sane.org.uk
A mental health charity providing information and support to people with mental health problems.

Special Needs Network
157–159 Portland Road
Hucknall
Nottingham NG15 7SB
Helpline: 0115 956 4852
Website:
www.nottssnn.freeserve.co.uk/index.html
A charity for parents of children with OCD, throughout Nottingham.

Triumph Over Phobia (Top UK)
Development Director
PO Box 1831
Bath BA2 4YW
Tel: 01225 330353
Fax: 01225 469212
Website: www.triumphoverphobia.com
*A charity founded with the help of
Issac Marks and designed to
promote exposure therapy for
helping people with OCD and
phobias.*

**Young Minds – The Children's Mental
Health Charity**
102–108 Clerkenwell Road
London EC1M 5SA
Tel: 020 7336 8445
Fax: 020 7336 8446
Website: www.youngminds.org.uk
*A charity for providing information
to help young people.*

USA

Anafranil Information Hotline
c/o CIBA Geigy
    Pharmaceutical Co.
556 Morris Avenue
Summit
NJ 07901
*For information on clomipramine
(Anafranil).*

**Association for Advancement of
Behaviour Therapy**
15 West 36th Street
New York
NY 10018
Tel: (212) 279 7970
Website: www.aabt.org
*An association to promote
behaviour therapy and cognitive
therapy. Provides links to
therapists for people in the USA,
England, Switzerland, Canada and
Peru.*

Kahli-Duphar
PO Box 29560
Columbus
Ohio 43229-1177
For information on fluvoxamine.

Obsessive-Compulsive Foundation Inc.
337 Notch Hill Road
North Branford
CT 06471
Tel: (203) 315 2190
Fax: (203) 315 2196
Website: www.ocfoundation.org
*A non-profit-making patient
support organisation, that gives
help in starting local self-help
groups, and in getting into contact
with others who have OCD.
Children can find penpals of a
similar age who are also affected.
Also publishes a quarterly
newsletter.*

Australia

Obsessive Compulsive Neurosis Support Group
Room 318, Epworth Building
33 Pirie Street
Adelaide
SA 5000
Tel: 231 1588 or 362 6772
A long-established and active self-help group and social network for people with OCD throughout Australia. Many local branches.

Websites

Please note that website addresses change frequently. The ones given here were valid when the book went to press.

www.ability.org.uk/Obsessive_Compulsive_Disorder.html
Designed by the charity Ability to encourage people with various disorders, this site relates specifically to OCD.

www.anxietycare.org.uk/documents/OCD-causesonline.htm
A source, from the charity Anxiety Care, of some useful information about OCD.

www.booksites.net/toates
The website for the biological psychology book by Frederick Toates [see 'Publications'], it contains updates on the latest information on biological psychology.

www.class.co.uk
The Class Publishing website will soon include a section giving full references to the material used for this book, for anyone interested in researching further.

www.geonius.com/ocd
A website of no acknowledged group, this has links to OCD-help organisations in countries around the world.

www.iop.kcl.ac.uk/main/Mhealth/
OCDyoung/default.htm
A site designed for young people by the London Institute of Psychiatry, a place famous for research and treatment of OCD.

www.mentalhealth.com/icd/p22-an05.html
The site of an organisation called Internet Mental Health, this is a source of information on the nature of OCD.

www.ppphealthcare.co.uk/html/health/
ocd.htm
A useful source of information on OCD and its treatment, from the medical insurance company PPPHealthcare.

www.prodigy.nhs.uk
A general health-care advice system of the Department of Health.

www.sandwellmind.co.uk/pages/ocd.htm
A bookshop that lists many books on OCD.

www.swayhouse.co.uk/SpecialistDirectory/
ocd.htm
Lists specialist counsellors, therapists and practitioners of psychological medicine who specialise in OCD. Their orientation is various and broad; only those offering behavioural or cognitive treatments can be recommended for someone with OCD.

www.veale.co.uk/ocdinfo.html
The website of Dr David Veale. He is Chairman of Obsessive Action, a charity for people with OCD and body dysmorphic disorder and an accredited cognitive behaviour therapist.

www.wspsdocs.com
A website for Western Suffolk Psychological Services, Huntington, NY, USA, the institution with which Fred Penzel [see 'Publications' entry] is associated.

Index

Have you found *Obsessive Compulsive Disorder* useful and practical? If so, you may be interested in these other titles from Class Publishing.

The '*at your fingertips*' series:

'Woe betide any clinicians or nurses whose patients have read this invaluable source of down-to-earth information when they have not.'
The Lancet

Our best selling series, the '*at your fingertips*' guides seek to help those who, having been diagnosed with a condition, have countless questions that need answering. These essential handbooks answer all the questions that those affected want to know about their health and condition.

The formula for the series follows a question-and-answer format, with real questions from sufferers and their families answered by medical experts at the top of their profession, in straightforward, jargon-free language. All these books are packed full of practical information for both patients and their families and friends.

Each title is only £14.99 plus £3 p&p. Topics covered range from diagnosis to treatment, and from relationships to welfare entitlements.

'Contains the answers the doctor wishes he had given if only he'd had the time.'
Dr Thomas Stuttaford, *The Times*

Titles currently available:

Acne • Allergies • Asthma • Beating Depression • Cancer • Dementia
Diabetes • Epilepsy • Heart Health • High Blood Pressure
Kidney Dialysis & Transplants • Multiple Sclerosis • Parkinson's
Psoriasis • Stroke

To order any of these titles in the '*at your fingertips*' series, please contact our Priority Order Service line on **01752 202 301**

Beating Depression – the 'at your fingertips' guide
NEW! £14.99
Dr Stefan Cembrowicz and Dr Dorcas Kingham

'A sympathetic and understanding guide for those people who experience depression.'
Marjorie Wallace, Chief Executive, SANE

Depression is one of the most common illnesses in the world – affecting up to one in five people at some time in their lives. Eminently treatable, the symptoms are more than just feeling down for a while; they range from tiredness and low mood, through to disturbed sleep and feelings of shame and inadequacy, even the wish to harm oneself.

Beating Depression – the 'at your fingertips' guide contains over 210 clear and helpful answers to questions actually asked by people with depression and their families. It gives you techniques for dealing with common symptoms, such as insomnia, agitation, panic and apathy, and contains details of where to go for further help and support. If you have any questions about depression, about medications and treatments, about self-help, about benefits and finance, and about where to turn for help and support – you will find the answers here.

'This is a very good, comprehensive book that is easy to use and follow. This is a book that, when read from cover to cover, can provide a comprehensive overview of depression, but can also be kept to hand and dipped into whenever the need arises.'
Amelia Mustapha, Depression Alliance

Positive Action for Health and Wellbeing
– the complete programme
£29.99
Dr Brian Roet

The complete step-by-step programme to take control of your life and your health.

'Over the years I have read countless self-help books and none of them helped. I started to read this book and could identify with most of the clients. No other book has ever had this effect on me.'

In this fascinating and original programme, Dr Brian Roet explains simply and clearly about the positive steps you can take to promote your own health and wellbeing. Using straightforward, easy and effective methods, the author shows you tried and tested steps to better health and self-esteem. Armed with this encouraging and empowering programme, you can overcome difficult problems, alleviate pain, reduce stress and tackle any fears and phobias you may have.

The complete guide comes in a presentation boxed set and contains:

- A practical guide – 272 pages that offer the key to solving long-term problems, whether physical, social or emotional.

- Your progress diary – in this personal progress diary, Dr Roet helps you to take positive steps to promote your own health and wellbeing.

- Double cassette pack – these tapes reinforce the practical messages. Listen to them as you work through the programme and they will show you how to put what you have learned into practice.

'I would like to say how much I have benefited from reading this book. I find it very helpful. This is the first time since my wife's death that I have actually told anyone how I feel.'

PRIORITY ORDER FORM

Cut out or photocopy this form and send it (*post free in the UK*) to:

Class Publishing Priority Service   Tel: **(01752) 202301**
FREEPOST (PAM 6219)
Plymouth PL6 7ZZ   Fax: **(01752) 202333**

Please send me urgently (*tick boxes below*)

		Post included price per copy (UK only)
☐	**Obsessive Compulsive Disorder** (ISBN 1 85959 069 1)	£17.99
☐	**Beating Depression – the 'at your fingertips' guide** (ISBN 1 85959 062 3)	£17.99
☐	**Positive Action for Health and Wellbeing – the complete programme** (ISBN 1 85959 041 1)	£32.99

TOTAL _____

For any of the other *'at your fingertips'* guides £17.99
Contact our Priority Order Service line on **01752 202 301**

Easy ways to pay

Cheque: I enclose a cheque payable to Class Publishing for £ _____

Credit card: Please debit my   ☐ Access   ☐ Visa   ☐ Amex   ☐ Switch

Number _____   Expiry date   / _____

Name _____

My address for delivery is _____

_____

Town _____   County _____   Postcode _____

Telephone number (*in case of query*) _____

Credit card billing address if different from above _____

_____

Town _____   County _____   Postcode _____

Class Publishing's guarantee: Remember that if, for any reason, you are not satisfied with these books, we will refund all your money, without any questions asked. Prices and VAT rates may be altered for reasons beyond our control.